"*Closer Together* tackles many of the essential questions that we each must face as we strive to create better lives. With refreshing candour and curiosity, Sophie Grégoire Trudeau draws on current research, interviews with experts, and the hard-won lessons she has learned herself to identify practical steps we can take to help ourselves to become happier and healthier."

—**Gretchen Rubin**, author of *Life in Five Senses*

"The heartfelt stories and insightful interviews in *Closer Together* are a call to action for openness, vulnerability, and radical self-acceptance—all of us can learn from Sophie Grégoire Trudeau's commitment to collective growth."

—**Arianna Huffington**, Founder & CEO, Thrive Global

"In *Closer Together* Sophie Grégoire Trudeau sparks an important conversation that a divided world needs more than ever. What's more, her warm and lively voice will make you feel as though you're having that conversation with an old friend."   —**Mark Critch**, author of *Son of a Critch*

"The wisdom contained in this book will move you to transform your brain and your life. *Closer Together* is an extraordinarily empathetic investigation of what our world needs now. With her unique brand of indefatigable charm and wit, Sophie casts a spell on the reader, wrapping them in a blanket of optimism. Read this book carefully, and it will feel like it's also reading you. Prepare for your heart to open and your soul to ripen."

—**Liz Plank**, author of *For the Love of Men*

"In *Closer Together* Sophie Grégoire Trudeau blends personal experiences with expert insights to offer smart, sensitive guidance on how to cultivate mental health, physical health, and our all-important relationships."

—**Lisa Damour**, PhD, author of *The Emotional Lives of Teenagers*

"This insightful book is a warm, wise, and generous exploration of getting to know ourselves better. By learning to face our past and embrace the contradictions and complexities of our human condition, *Closer Together* shows us how we can live our lives with courage, authenticity, and joy."

—**Sara Kuburic**, author of *It's On Me*

Closer Together

KNOWING OURSELVES, LOVING EACH OTHER

Sophie Grégoire Trudeau

RANDOM HOUSE CANADA

Excerpt from *Attached: The New Science of Adult Attachment and How It Can
Help You Find—and Keep—Love* by Amir Levine, M.D., and Rachel S. F. Heller, M.A.,
copyright © 2010 by Amir Levine and Rachel Heller. Used by permission of Tarcher,
an imprint of Penguin Publishing Group, a division of Penguin Random House LLC.
All rights reserved.

Image of vagus nerve on page 247 used under licence from Shutterstock.com.
All other images courtesy of the author.

Library and Archives Canada Cataloguing in Publication

Title: Closer together : knowing ourselves, loving each other / Sophie Grégoire Trudeau.
Names: Grégoire Trudeau, Sophie, author.
Identifiers: Canadiana (print) 20230439845 | Canadiana (ebook) 2023043990X |
ISBN 9781039007444 (hardcover) | ISBN 9781039007451 (EPUB)
Subjects: LCSH: Self-actualization (Psychology) | LCSH: Mental health. |
LCSH: Grégoire Trudeau, Sophie.
Classification: LCC BF637.S4 G74 2024 | DDC 158.1—dc23

Book design: Lisa Jager
Jacket photography: Wade Hudson
Printed in Canada

2 4 6 8 9 7 5 3

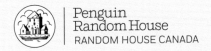

*I dedicate this book to every being who has loved me and whom
I loved in return. You showed me the way within.*

Contents

All human beings are united by birth, life, death,

and every emotion in between. YUNG PUEBLO

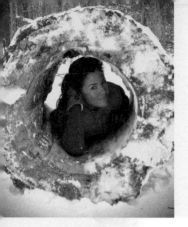

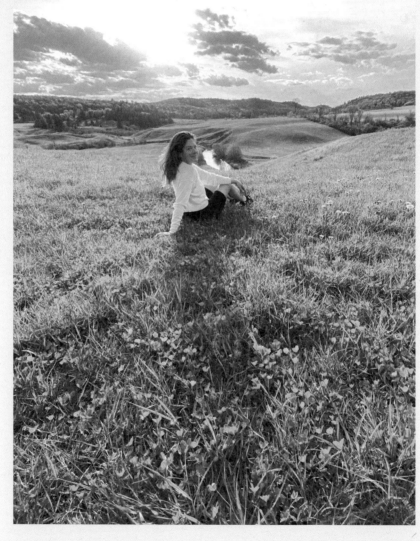

Introduction

Holding Ourselves

Remember always that you have not only the right to be
an individual; you have an obligation to be one. You cannot make
any useful contribution in life unless you do this.

ELEANOR ROOSEVELT

Let's start with a tiny confession—there will be more to come.
There's this thing I do every time I find myself standing around
somewhere: in a line at the supermarket when someone is taking
forever to place their items on the conveyor belt at the checkout,
or standing at a function, maybe, or waiting offstage before I'm
announced to make a speech. I also noticed myself doing it while I
was sitting at my desk for months writing this book (when I wasn't
occasionally doing jumping jacks to get the feeling back into my
legs!). It's subtle—if you looked at me, you wouldn't even be able to
tell, unless you were really observing closely, which I hope you were

not! First, I root my feet deeper into the floor, which supports me. Then I try to find where my breath is in my body; I make it deeper and longer, and more spacious in my belly than in my chest. Next, I check if my shoulders are too close to my ears and release them. And last, whether I'm standing upright or sitting in front of the computer, comes the pelvic tilt, where I push my hips a tiny bit forward and bring my tailbone down toward the floor. All of a sudden, I feel more grounded, solid, and calm.

I've always been curious about how people inhabit their bodies. As a child, I could effortlessly pick up on facial expressions and cues, any quirks in posture or tone of voice or tics. Once back in the privacy of my bedroom, I would attempt to imitate their stances or movements (surprise, surprise—my kids pick up on the same stuff!). Ever since I studied yoga in my thirties, and became an occasional teacher, I have had a natural, loving desire to adjust the skeletal positioning of human bodies around me. If you've ever attended a yoga class and have given consent to hands-on adjustments, you'll know what I mean. A beautiful assist while you are sitting on your mat: the teacher takes both hands to roll your shoulders back and then elongate your neck by softly lifting up your head. Sometimes that's all it takes to feel more relaxed, to bring out a sigh of relief.

Did you maybe adjust your own body a tiny bit while reading this?

There's no question that I am deeply interested in physical alignment, which can offer hints as to mood, health, disease, personality, and energy. The way we walk, sit, or stand can reflect habits, a former injury, and our own fitness level. But I'm also fundamentally and passionately curious about another type of alignment: our unique *emotional* alignment. In fact, that's why I decided to write this book.

As a mental health, emotional literacy, and gender equality advocate for the past two decades, I've discovered more about human emotions than I ever thought I would. As much as we are thinking beings, we are *feeling* and *sensing* beings at our core. Whether we feel happy and hopeful or angry and fearful, we engage not only in a physical or facial expression but also in an emotional posture. Are we truly aware of this process and of how we hold ourselves from the inside? Do we observe, strengthen, and stretch the parts of ourselves, and our minds, that need it the most?

Tell me: If you were to take a snapshot of your mental landscape, what would it look like? Whatever lights and shadows you can discern, whatever moods, emotions, and images, know that they are all part of you. Much of what you've seen or felt was wired into what we call your "primitive brain" during childhood, through your relationship with your parent or caretaker. You carried this hard-wiring through your childhood and into your teenage years (whether rebellious or not), and through the emotional discoveries you made as you grew into your adult life. We tend to convince ourselves that we are unique—so very different from everyone else around us. But the truth of the matter is that the structure of our brains hasn't changed in more than two hundred thousand years. Where we differ is in our programming, which is dependent on the care we received, the relationships we foster, and the experiences we live through. As therapist and author Vienna Pharaon explains in *The Origins of You*, "understanding your origin wound and the long-standing destructive patterns it leads to will go a long way to addressing conflicts and behaviours that trouble you today." If you're doubting that your childhood experiences affect how you come into relationship with others and yourself, then, just like me, you'll be surprised by what you'll learn in this book.

Twenty years ago, when I was a young radio and television host in Quebec—a newcomer in my field—I decided to speak out about my struggles with an eating disorder. It wasn't an easy decision. I was hesitant to show my vulnerability publicly and wondered if I would ever be hired again. No one spoke much about mental health back then, and especially not about eating disorders. But deep down, I felt like it was the right thing to do. I faced my fear and went ahead with it—and it became a turning point that has given my life direction.

Suffering is part of life. We don't need to avoid or transcend it. Rather, we must develop wisdom, self-reliance, and resilience *through* and *with* our pain. In our search for happiness, we must uncover its roots, as we carry them with us into our mental state and, therefore, into whatever we do and whomever we come into relationship with. Yale psychology professor Laurie R. Santos, who has studied the science of happiness, found that many of us are working at and doing things that actually put a damper on our level of happy. "Natural selection isn't into us being happy," she said in a *Time* magazine interview, in which she discussed her own experience with burnout during the pandemic years. "It would prefer we drove ourselves into the ground trying to survive, reproduce, and get the most resources. It's not in it for joy."

Think about that for a minute: on a purely neurological level, our brains don't care if we're happy. *We* need to make that happen, and running ourselves ragged as we chase good grades, status, titles, eternal youth, and bliss isn't going to do it.

It actually takes courage and work to be happy. We must learn to live with integrity and coherence, staying true to our values and expressing our authentic self. In this way, we can take control over ourselves and our lives. As Dr. Santos says: "Getting out of our own way is the first step to happiness!"

I'm still learning how to get out of my own way. Discovering more about the intricacies of my inner wiring and emotional posture, my childhood, the defence mechanisms I've developed, my ongoing longing for safety, and so much more, has allowed me to better understand why I suffered from an eating disorder, how I could heal from it, and how to live with and accept the suffering that had led to it. And along the way, I'm transforming my life—and my brain—with every step.

In November 2022, the world population hit eight billion. That's eight billion lives, eight billion minds, eight billion hearts. There's a lot of thinking and feeling taking place on planet Earth.

Unfortunately, the World Health Organization tells us that one out of every eight people suffers from a mental health disorder, and mental health is the single-biggest contributor to years lost at work because of disability. And let's remember that a healthy mind is not simply the absence of a mental illness. None of us should have to suffer alone.

But before we start pathologizing ourselves, we must also be more aware of the societal structures in which we live. Critical world problems, disparity, gender inequality, climate change, and the incessant flow of news and knowledge being bulldozed our way every day are all examples of environmental factors that can deeply affect our well-being.

It's time for us to stop spinning and to be more aware of *why* we feel and think the way we do, and why so many of us find ways to numb our pain.

Through the years, I've had the privilege of meeting people from all walks of life, each with their own unique stories of loss, triumph, heartache, and mind ache. From world-renowned actors, rock stars, writers, and artists to world leaders, queens and kings, Nobel Prize winners, and activists, every being I've encountered has their own emotional struggles. And it makes no difference whether they have a big title beside their name or no title at all. I have also observed that we are all one trauma away from each other. The homeless person you pass on the street, for example? That could be you or me after trauma. It takes just a single dramatic life event or a series of smaller traumas to affect our nervous system and brain. This is our shared truth.

My truth is that I'm reaching out to you, in my late forties, as a mother of three, a woman, a friend, a partner, a sister, and a trustworthy, vulnerable, and courageous ally. I want us to take steps and risks together, on our parallel paths, so we can find our light-filled purpose. The goal of understanding and healing ourselves belongs to all of us, and depends on all of us.

British-Canadian physician and psychiatrist Dr. Kwame McKenzie describes *mental health* as a term that refers to our emotional, psychological, and social well-being. It affects how we feel, think, and act. Every facet of our lives and every role we have (be it as a child, parent, partner, worker, friend, community member, or elder) is impacted by our mental health. In Canada alone, mental illness costs the country an estimated $50 billion a year. Most people who die by suicide are considered to have mental illness, which also increases one's risk for diabetes, heart problems, and high blood pressure, to name just a few. "Many people would say that stigma and prejudice are the reasons we do not value mental illness," Dr. McKenzie says. "The myth is that mental illnesses reflect a character flaw and that we should be able to pull ourselves out of it."

This myth is a tough one to eradicate. Knowing that, we must work harder at destigmatizing mental disorders by better understanding how we function physiologically and psychologically. In itself, this renewed awareness decreases our stress levels. More of that, please!

This outlook is where the concept of emotional intelligence (known as EQ, or emotional quotient) takes its deepest meaning. Dr. McKenzie tells us that individuals, companies, and countries with high levels of emotional intelligence outperform those with lower levels. But low levels of mental health undermine the ability of both high levels of IQ (intellectual quotient) and EQ to have the desired impact. "'Mental capital' is considered a capital because we can invest in it and grow it," he told me. "It will then act as a resource for us. But if we do not look after it and invest in it, then it could shrink."

All of the fascinating collaborators I've interviewed for this book have worked hard to look after and invest in our shared mental capital. They've studied in depth our human capacity for optimized health and psychological flexibility. In these pages, you will meet some of the best and brightest minds in the fields of mental health and well-being: child psychologists, neuroscientists, addiction specialists, relationship experts, artists, mindfulness teachers, and more. I've been so blessed to speak with them and have done so with the goal of making their incredible knowledge and insight more accessible to all of us—as it should be. Think about it: we teach our kids how to read and count, but wouldn't it be nice if they had access at an early age to what I call a "universal emotional library"—a space within themselves that they could draw from when they felt down, confused, angry, or more? This library would hold a common vocabulary and emotional encyclopedia, ready to help us learn more about our emotions and how to sit with our pain in a calmer way. Imagine what kind of world it would be if all the adults you know had a full view of their emotional posture and had learned to regulate their own emotions. That includes you and me. Working in this way toward more self-awareness and compassion would give us greater agency over ourselves and build a collective resilience and a sense of togetherness, which can, in turn, help us confront what we are facing as human beings in this day and age.

This is why I wrote this book; it is my humble contribution to that goal. It takes us on a journey through our emotional landscape—from childhood to adulthood, with some stops in between. It explores why we feel and think the way we do, and the ways in which we can change those feelings and thoughts for the better. Here are just a few of the crucial questions we'll answer:

- How does our childhood bond of attachment continue to affect us throughout our life, and especially in our relationships?
- What are the challenges of coming of age in our go-go-go culture?
- How can we find our passion and purpose?
- How can knowing ourselves transform our friendships and loving relationships?
- What tools do we have at hand to deal with big emotions and trauma?
- How do sleep, nutrition, exercise, creativity, mindfulness, and a sense of playfulness contribute to our mental health and sense of well-being?

Whether you're single or married, a teenager or a mid-lifer or older, a parent or not, you are welcomed on this journey. Embark with me. I won't kid you; it's going to be an intense ride. But it sure won't be boring. The warrior and lover in me knows that taking risks and cultivating self-respect is a rebellious, mischievous, and loving act. We must develop more faith in ourselves. But first, we must understand our own emotional history and change the patterns that have come before us, the ones that are holding us back in ways we often don't even realize. Our world is calling on us to be the breakers of these cycles of negativity!

When I mentioned this idea to bestselling author Terry Real, whom you might have seen on Oprah Winfrey's show, and whom we will hear more from later, he agreed, saying, "Family pathology rolls from generation to generation, taking down everything in its path, until one person in one generation has the courage to turn to face it. That person brings peace to their ancestors and spares the children that follow. And that's the work. And beyond that, your family pathology is situated inside a cultural background: the culture of patriarchy, the culture of racism, the culture of misogyny, the culture of toxic individualism."

We are going to be facing some soft and hard truths together. Get ready. You might feel shocked, surprised, disappointed, sad, or angry, or maybe even inspired and profoundly reassured as you explore your emotional landscape. It doesn't really matter how you navigate the path that winds through these pages. What counts is that you *feel*. Fully. Often, it is when we reach our lowest points that we face our truth. And it hurts. Wherever you are in your life right now, know that every day can be a new beginning. We can rewire our brains and mend our hearts. It's all possible, but it's not easy. And it shouldn't be. But together, we meet in ways that can help us heal and cope, no matter what struggles we are facing individually. And as bestselling author and psychotherapist Esther Perel writes: "The quality of our relationships determines the quality of our lives."

In a world that is constantly trying to define us, we must know ourselves better in order to resist those pressures and bloom into our authentic selves. Feeling makes us human, and being human makes us feel. Let's come closer to knowing ourselves so we can love each other better.

Part 1

Foundations

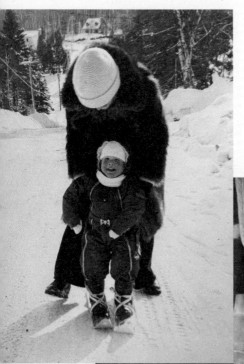

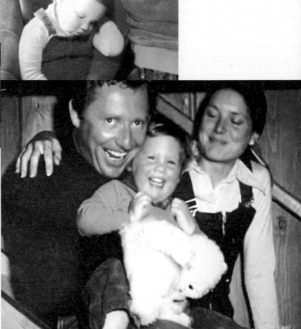

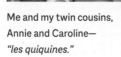

Me and my twin cousins,
Annie and Caroline—
"les quiquines."

Setting Roots

Childhood, Attachment, and Where It All Starts

Genius is no more than childhood recaptured at will,

childhood equipped now with man's physical means to express itself . . .

CHARLES BAUDELAIRE

Montreal, April 24, 1975. It's very early morning. My mother, who suffered twice from tuberculosis, once in her youth and once in adulthood, and who had been told that having children might be a problem, is in full contractions, ready to birth her first (and only) baby. My dad, Jean, is with her in the delivery room. There's no time for an epidural, and my beautiful mom, a nurse herself, is giving her all through the pain and exhaustion. In an attempt to encourage her, my Type-A-personality dad says, "Estelle, your head is going to explode! Stop pushing from your face and start pushing from your ass!"

Understandably impatient, and purple-red, my mom gives him *the look*. (In her position, I probably would have screamed at him, or worse.) The whole process takes about four hours, and, finally, here I am. I'm cone-headed, thanks to the use of forceps, and reddish-blue from a lack of oxygen, so my dad—who had worked as a first-aid responder years before—points to the incubator and says, "She's cold and she needs air! Quick, put her in the barbecue!"

I'm laughing as I write this, picturing the scene. It's such a perfect glimpse into my lovely, dear, beautiful, and wacky family—the family that gave me so much and played such a huge part in shaping the person I am today.

This is true for all of us, isn't it? A big part of who we are is shaped in the early years of our life, and we carry that sense of self with us into adulthood. And the older we get, the harder it is to go back to who we are at our core. Too often, we get defined by our looks, our job titles (or lack thereof), who we follow or don't follow on social media and how many we are followed by ourselves, our socio-economic status, where or how we pray, whom we hang out with, or whom we marry. It often happens in the blink of an eye, based on nothing more than what is obvious on the surface.

I've experienced so many different versions of this "quick assessment" in my life—especially over the last several years. At first glance, a person who's come up to me on the street or at a restaurant may recognize me as someone they see now and again on their television or in the newspaper, wearing formal clothes that don't represent the real me, only the me that attends an official event every so often. Sometimes I'd be asked if I was "Trudeau's wife," to which I usually responded with a grin: "Well actually, I'm Sophie—pleased to meet you!" While that typically elicited a giggle, what I always hoped for was a more profound connection.

Although I don't think we should define ourselves through specific words, since they can't encompass an entire human nature and personality, I would say that I see myself as a passionate, creative, and courageous woman, a hands-on, present, deeply loving mother, a devoted daughter, an intrepid sportswoman (according to a friend, the more appropriate term is *breakneck*), a loyal friend, a fierce advocate, and a steadfast ally—someone who has experienced joy and sadness and triumphs and challenges and all of the messy, wonderful things that make up our lives. In other words, I'm a fully formed human being, just like you.

And yet how often do we look deeper, for something that is more real? So much of what floats on the surface these days stands for nothing, and yet we form perceptions and even make decisions based on them, rather than on deeper truths. If we're being honest, how often do we go there even in relation to ourselves? Because facing our truth is hard, as individuals and as a society. But knowing who we are is the first step toward living a life that is whole and healthy and deeply authentic. When we know ourselves in this way, we are so much better prepared to meet others on these same terms, to build strong and emotional connections that recognize our similarities and respect and celebrate our differences. That's a pretty good motivation for some self-examination.

As I mentioned in the introduction, I've been an advocate for mental health and well-being for more than two decades now. I've also done a lot of exploring when it comes to the emotional hard-wiring from childhood that has made me the person I've grown into. One of the most amazing things I've learned is just how important our first few years are when it comes to forming the peaks and valleys of our emotional landscape. These early days in our lives really do set the tone for all that follows; vital clues about who we really are deep down inside are hidden there, if only we decide to look.

Early Days

I'll break the ice. Here's something I know about myself: for as long as I can remember, I've had a deep need for authentic connection. Years ago, I attended a father-daughter event with Justin and Ella-Grace to raise funds for the FitSpirit foundation, which encourages girls to get active. Because I was the foundation's ambassador, the girls knew about my personal struggles with eating disorders. While my daughter and her father made their way to the dance floor, a young girl and her father walked over to me to chat. When her father's attention momentarily shifted away, the young woman leaned in and whispered in my ear, "My dad doesn't know, but I'm not doing well, and I have an eating disorder." I held her tight against me as I tried to hold back my tears. I told her that what she'd done just by telling me was so courageous, and that she'd actually taken a huge first step. I also let her know how beneficial it would be to her healing if she let her dad know what she was going through.

Over the years, I've come to understand why encounters like this are so precious to me, and why I revel in the safe and trusting feeling that comes with authentic connection. And yup, it all goes right back to my childhood, to those early days when the contours of my emotional landscape were taking shape.

I grew up in nature in the small Laurentian town of Sainte-Adèle, Quebec, up until I was four years old. We first lived in a brown and white wooden cabin that we shared on weekends and in the summers with my paternal aunt and uncle. If you had known me then, you would have probably noted a sense of curiosity, laughter, mischievousness, and intrepidness, but also some sadness. Thanks to my dad's and uncle's love of photography, many pictures were taken during these years, mostly of me alone in the forest, scruffily dressed, hands in dirt, hair tousled, playing with squirrels and wildlife, camping, swimming in the lake, sitting by a campfire, reading, or showing off my ballet and sports moves, my chubby face squeezed by loving hands or licked by my dog Nikon, who one day disappeared without a trace. I'm told I was a deeply sensitive, empathetic, creative, and romantic little being. Whining was not welcome in my household, so I learned to switch from one emotional state to another rapidly, and to not hold grudges.

Back then, my happy places were the forest and water—and they still are. I clearly recall feeling that my connection to animals and trees was magical and unique, and that I shared a secret language with them, one that transcended words. I believed I could understand the whispers of the wind and confide to the trees my deepest secrets, which would be stored forever under thick and craggy bark. I felt naturally tethered to the Earth. I loved and respected her, and she loved me in return. It was such a safe and vast place to be. Canadian painter Emily Carr described this state so blissfully: "So still were the big woods where I sat, sound might not yet have been born." In many ways, the adults who introduced me to life encouraged my natural propensity to be close to nature and attentive to her soft or harsh moods, which changed depending on the lessons she needed us to learn. I spent a good deal of time alone, so I also developed a peaceful sense of solitude that could turn to loneliness at times.

I dreamed of having siblings to play with, because I spent most of my time imagining games and scenarios by myself. Like most only children, I felt pressure in different ways to fulfill all of my parents' needs and expectations while also being at the centre of their dynamics. They were both kind, sensitive, funny, cultivated, curious, and outgoing people, but I clearly remember my parents fighting and my mom often being sad. I used to lie in my bed at night trying not to hear and feel the tension from their harsh words, trying not to feel the pain, trying to settle my attention elsewhere. I was so grateful for the comfort of Snowball, the kitten my parents gave me when I was about six. He looked more like a little cotton ball when I got him. It felt as if my heart soared to the sky when I got him (and it sank heavily back to earth two decades later, when he died a few months after I moved out of my parents' house).

Although my father and mother had their difficulties, my father was extremely affectionate with me, giving out huge kisses and cuddling with me in bed in the early morning. My mom was more inclined toward a soft embrace. I longed to sit beside her in the brown corduroy chair she would read in for hours, and I hold on dearly to the only picture of a moment like that that remains—saved after our basement flooded in Montreal in 2013 and Justin and I lost many of our child-hood pictures (this is why I wanted to share it with you at the beginning of this chapter).

My parents were my first influences, my role models, my earliest loves. My father, Jean Grégoire, is my philosopher and sporadic life coach. A francophone born and raised in Hull, Quebec, he spent his summers in Shawinigan, Lac des Piles, and Blue Sea Lake. An ethical and hard worker, he built his career from small-town bank teller to account manager and successful stockbroker as he moved us from the countryside into Montreal. He has a wicked sense of humour and was the life of the party and a mischievous trick player (I inherited that trait from him). Sensitive, witty, and very intense, he made me chop wood with an axe before I was ten, had me pulling soaked logs from frozen winter lakes, and taught me how to water-ski bare-foot, downhill ski, and drive boats and snowmobiles. Most importantly, my dad passed on to me his own love of nature. When I was about five, he taught me to taste and identify different pine needles with my eyes closed. He and his brother, Marc Grégoire, a former water-ski champion and marketing whiz, would pull me on a sleigh while snowshoeing or cross-country skiing, returning home only late in the evening to my very worried mom. He would ask me to lay my ears on rocks and listen to the "sound of silence." I still catch myself doing it, or I'll invite my kids to do the same. I'm usually rewarded with a couple of eye rolls, but the calm feeling it brings is well worth whatever ribbing I get.

Spending quality time with my dad at an early age profoundly developed my five senses and my personality. We played in nature together, as she was the ultimate guiding Mother. We learned from her all the time. My dad referred to Mother Nature as his muse and "le parfum ultime." To this day, I'm colourfully inspired by sight (I paint) and I'll dance to almost any sound (I play a little piano, flute, and guitar). When the wind touches my neck, I shiver (I'm a passionate lover). My palate is always in search of new experiences (I love to cook and I'm a foodie), and don't even start me on scents (I almost chose to study at Cinquième Sens in France after reading Patrick Süskind's *Perfume*). It is also because of my father—and my own courageous nature—that I love to surf, scuba dive with sharks, alpine ski in scary terrain at crazy speed, and jump out of an airplane, parachuting in tandem at fourteen thousand feet. You name it; I'm probably willing to try it. I'm not without fear, but I still go for it. My nickname used to be *"La Tornade,"* since I never stopped pushing and exploring, and wanted everyone around me to push their own boundaries as well. My poor friends! I've calmed down since I was young. A bit.

My mother, Estelle, is a former nurse who worked mostly with psychiatric patients. From my earliest days, she surrounded me with arts, literature, fashion, and beauty. We cooked, we read, we danced, we confided, and we went on long walks (we still do, and from behind, we are easily mistaken for each other, because we have a similar body and strut). We share a passion for the French language and francophone culture from Quebec and France. She ignited my lasting love of writing and poetry, and she fostered my love of music by sharing her own fondness of all its forms with me, from rock to opera and everything in between. Like my father, she loves the outdoors. She would often pull me on a sleigh to daycare in big snowstorms. I would whine and tell her I just wanted to take the car. She'd remind me that my dad had to use our car to drive to work, and that the sleigh was the perfect way to get some fresh air. I've now done the exact same thing with my kids. I have incredible pictures of me and my mom—wearing snowsuits and goggles in the midst of a snowfall—pulling the kids to daycare along the city streets. The apple truly doesn't fall far from the tree!

My parents and I moved to Montreal after I turned four. I missed the countryside, but the time I'd spent there left a beautiful, indelible mark on my mind, body, and heart. It grounded me, and I carried it with me as I explored my new surroundings with curiosity.

I was also interested in the world of adults. Once, while on a trip together, my parents and I were in our bathing suits, watching the sun set. At some point, they turned around and realized I was gone. Before launching into a full-fledged panic, they searched the resort and found me sitting in the middle of a hot tub, chatting away with a group of adults. They got a good laugh out of that one. Maybe I was subliminally getting back at them for the time they went on their first "child-free" vacation. I was about three years old and I stayed at the house of a close friend, but I still remember feeling sad. I sat in a rocking chair with tears rolling down my cheeks for hours every day. With my family unit being as small as it was, I felt even more alone than usual when my parents were gone.

It's not surprising, really, that I loved any occasion when we got to see extended family. Sunday evenings were magic. That's when my twin cousins, Annie and Caroline (whom I held in my arms as newborns and warmly referred to as "*les quiquines*," a word I invented and that has no translation in English), would come for a family dinner. This communal meal made me feel as if I were part of a "normal" family, with life all around and in the house.

As I mentioned near the beginning of this chapter, when I go back into my sensory and emotional memory, I do remember feeling lonely. I recall being continuously in tune with my parents' emotional states, often trying to uplift my mom as I sensed her sadness, and trying both to match my dad's very social and high-alert attitude and understand his complete emotional absence. I knew he loved me, but we didn't spend much quality time together. One winter, when we were at the cottage we rented on weekends in Sainte-Adèle, I really wanted to build a snow fort. I kept asking my dad to come help, and for a few minutes he did, but then I was left to build it on my own for the rest of the weekend. I'm sure this has happened to a lot of kids, but I often felt hurt and abandoned by his behaviour, which repeated itself in different "micro" forms through the years. He would tell me he loved me and encourage me to follow my passions, but more and more, he withdrew into his own world. In a way, I had to grieve the hero and mentor I'd found in him.

I've since come to understand he was suffering in his own ways—he'd experienced his own family trauma and loss, including from the aftermath of a tragic boating accident that took place when he was a young adult—but back then, I had no idea what was keeping my dad emotionally distant. As in every family, we all had our own issues and battles. Many of my family members, on both sides, suffered from addiction, alcoholism, depression, anger, and verbal abuse. As a child and as a teenager, I was witness to some of it.

But there was so much joy, too. I liked school and studied quite hard. I made friends, attended summer camp, and enjoyed the company of boys—A LOT. When I was about five years old, I was actually convinced I was going to marry famous Quebec singer René Simard one day. I would stare at his album cover and press my lips against it, pretending to kiss him (I did this a bit later on with George Michael's CDs, too).

When I wasn't daydreaming about pop stars or the boys I actually knew, I spent time playing in the new pool my parents had built in our yard. I was in heaven. During the summer months, I would spend hours practising my dives and playing mermaid by myself, until my dad would surreptitiously approach with the huge hose he used to fill up the pool. He would aim the extremely powerful jet at me to start a funny game of hide-and-seek. Come to think of it, this is probably how I learned to hold my breath for so long. These little episodes of laughter reminded me of how naturally we knew how to be playful together, even if these moments were too rare for my needs.

After second grade, when I was around eight years old, my parents decided to send me to a large private school in Outremont. Mont-Jésus-Marie was a fifteen-minute drive from our home, but a long way from our neighbourhood. Leaving my group of friends was a shock, but I'd been taught and encouraged to adapt to change, and so I went along with it. But the transition was not seamless. Apart from my good friend Annie, who moved from Saint-Clément at the same time, I did not know whom to hang out with. For the first weeks, and perhaps months, I spent countless recess breaks alone in the schoolyard, looking out into a forest that led to a mountain. I remember befriending the air, the trees, the leaves that surrounded me, as I had in my younger years. They were a natural solace. I carried sadness within me for quite a while and would come home from school crying, with no one but my mom to share it with. She would hold me in her arms and try to reassure me as best she could.

Slowly but surely, though, friendship and love found their way into my life. I began to play Ping-Pong in the recreation room with some of the boys, including Michel (Miche) Trudeau, Justin's younger brother, who tragically lost his life in an avalanche when he was only twenty-three. Christine and Nathalie brought me into their circle (and we remain the best of friends today), and I developed an overwhelming crush on a boy named Frédéric. He was a year older than I was, short and athletic, with an angelic face. Our homes were a kilometre apart, and we hung out together after school, riding our bikes, and took pottery classes at the local community centre. We wrote each other love letters, a few of which I think I still have, and Fred would put some of his allowance quarters in them, along with a hidden-words game where the missing words formed the sentence "I love you." I cherish these memories.

Once or twice a year, the fourth- and fifth-grade students would walk in a line through the dimly lit hallways with their creaking floors to visit the coffin of Mother Marie-Rose Eulalie Durocher (1811-1849), the founder and first superior of the Sisters of the Holy Names of Jesus and Mary in Canada. We had to keep silent when we entered that room, and a certain gloom hung in the air. Sometimes we went on into la Grande Chapelle, one of the most beautiful rooms I had ever seen. The choir we were all a part of as pupils sounded its best under the giant painted dome. During Mass, incense adorned the air, an organ played elegantly, and I knew all the prayers and songs by heart. Unfortunately, it wasn't uncommon for a couple of students to faint as the air became smoky and boredom set in! I still carry with me the colours, shapes, sounds, and emotions I experienced and felt in that chapel, even though my relationship with religion and the Catholic Church has changed over the years. In many ways, the feeling I got from being at peace in and with nature was also found there. Growing up in nature at a young age made me feel and believe in something bigger than what the eye could see. I felt like that force, energy, divine presence, or whatever you long to call it surrounded all of us and was somehow within all of us, too.

These days, when things in my life get much more challenging than what people might typically imagine, I try to recollect that inner peace, that life force I felt when I was free, careless, and connected to the great outdoors as a child. This is why I still spend so much time out there today—because how I feel in that setting is who I am deep in my core. I revisit other rituals from that time in my life as well. My parents both went to bed early and rose with the sun, and taught me to do the same. To this day, there's nothing I love more than to get up when everyone else is sleeping, light a candle, and dwell in that familiar, comforting silence where I can gain perspective about who and what I am. Some things really do stay with you.

The Bonds of Attachment

I should probably revise that last sentence. When it comes to things we carry out of our childhoods and into our adult lives, more than *some* things stay with us. Traits like a fondness for rising early and a love of nature (in my case) tell only the very beginning of the story. Science is showing us that the quality and consistency of the physical and psychological care we received in the first months and years of our life—and the bond of attachment we formed with our parents or caregivers—are great determinants of how our brains are wired and what we consider to be our places of emotional safety.

When you stop and think about it, it makes perfect sense. All of us come into the world helpless, malleable, and vulnerable. We need adults to be attentive to our needs at almost every moment. In fact, our physical and emotional survival depends on it. If our basic needs are met as growing newborns and our relationship with our parent or caregiver is filled with consistency and quality care, we form a healthy team adept at what's known as "co-regulation"—a process in which both participants in a relationship are constantly adjusting their behaviours and interactions to maintain a positive and safe emotional state. If attention isn't paid and our needs aren't consistently met? Well, that can have a lasting impact on our lives.

In the 1950s and '60s, John Bowlby, a British psychologist, psychiatrist, and psychoanalyst, developed the "attachment theory" to describe the emotional bonds that exist between a mother (or primary caregiver) and her child and the ways in which our earliest relationships can set the tone for our psychological development. In order to thrive, young children need the adults in their lives to be deeply present; they need to be picked up, cared for, played with, and interacted with. They need connection. When that connection exists, a secure bond of attachment forms—a sense of safety and trust that carries into other relationships throughout the child's life. But if the adults in a child's life are not deeply present and willing and able to care for that child through soothing touch, gentle words, and consistent eye-to-eye contact—through consistent and authentic connection—the bonds of attachment could be anxious or avoidant, setting the stage for less trusting relationships in the future. (See the box on page 32 to learn more about the different attachment styles.)

Thanks to Bowlby and others who followed, we now know that the attachment bond we formed in our earliest years has a universal scientific resonance, from cradle to grave. It is our greatest common biological denominator. Can you recall your earliest memories of how your main caregiver interacted with you?

I learned more about this vital connection when I talked to one of the world's most respected attachment bond specialists, Dr. Allan Schore. For the past thirty years, he has written and expanded on modern attachment theory—a neurobiological update of Bowlby's seminal studies. His work was first presented in his pioneering 1994 book, *Affect Regulation and the Origin of the Self: The Neurobiology of Emotional Development.*

We're going to get into some science here, but stay with me; I promise it will be worth it. Allan explains that the early experiences between mother (or whichever caregiver is present) and baby are actually imprinted into the wiring of the baby's developing right brain, which takes charge when it comes to processing emotional and social information, and also the non-verbal communication of emotions between the mother's brain and the baby's. And guess what? These dynamics begin in the last trimester of pregnancy and continue right through the second year of life. It's a truly critical period of right-brain growth that takes place before the onset of a left-brain (cognitive functions and logic) growth spurt around age three.

In other words, when babies are born, the ventral vagal branch of the parasympathetic nervous system—which is part of the vagus nerve and works to relax the body after periods of stress or danger—is not fully refined. In order to achieve that refinement, and for us to learn to soothe ourselves, the ventral vagal branch must be used with good attunement and attachment. A caring relationship between mother and child activates this branch and can actually lower the heart rate. It's as if an unconscious yet synchronized brain-eye-touch-voice dance is happening between mother and baby, and we carry that rhythm with us into adulthood. (For more about how the parasympathetic nervous system works, see the box on page 26.)

When we spoke, I asked Allan how that rhythm shows up in our daily lives, where we receive emotional information and cues from the people we interact with. "The pacing of emotional information is much, much more rapid than verbal communication," he told me. "And when we're emotionally engaged with each other, my right brain picks up your facial expression in one hundred milliseconds. So, whatever your words are on top of that, at the gut level, I have read those other communications first. And that really is what's going to drive how close or distant we are. The first thing we pick up are the right-brain cues."

Fascinating, right? What Allan is telling us is that the "emotional music" we carry from our childhood provides the "soundtrack" of our relationships. If the melody contains notes of toxic stress, parental emotional unavailability, or violence, it lets us know we aren't secure. We may be anxious or afraid, and we may not trust others with our heart. With this music playing in our unconscious mind, we may be "dysregulated"; that is, lacking the emotional tools needed to deal with the ups and downs of relationships, to repair the little (and not-so-little) hurts and damages that come our way. And as Allan stresses, "chronic relational trauma without repair" can interfere with the growth of the right brain and could "predispose to later psychopathologies." But if the melody holds notes of intuition, vulnerability, and attunement, then it's telling us we are safe and secure. It gives us the biological tools we need to regulate our emotional experiences and deal with whatever comes our way, whether it's celebrating successes or repairing failures.

Our Nervous System at Work

Our autonomic (meaning "involuntary") nervous system controls so many of the body's functions—from breathing and heartbeat to circulation and blood pressure to metabolism and digestion. Among these functions and others, it works to achieve homeostasis, or a state in which our body is operating at an optimal and balanced level. To get the job done, it relies on two branches.

The primary function of the **sympathetic branch** is to stimulate the body's fight-or-flight response when presented with any potential danger. It does this by creating a state of alertness. You might notice dilated pupils, an increased heart rate, a lack of saliva, or an upset stomach.

The primary function of the **parasympathetic branch** is to stimulate the body's "rest and digest" and "feed and breed" responses. It wants to bring the body into a calm and composed state and stop it from overworking. When the parasympathetic branch is at work, you might notice a slower heartbeat, relaxed muscles, and calm digestive organs. The important vagus nerve, which we'll learn more about in chapter 9, is part of the para-sympathetic nervous system.

These two systems are constantly working together. In the coming chapters, we'll learn how to better influence this partner-ship by recognizing and dealing with the "go-to" default stress responses that were wired into our brains and bodies in our earliest years.

In his book *IntraConnected*, Dr. Daniel Siegel talks about this sense of security created in early childhood—when the child's imma-ture brain is using the mature circuits of the adult brain to regulate itself—as the basis for our capacity to connect, to belong within a "we" without losing the integrity of the "me." It's how we develop what researchers call "epistemic trust," which is a fancy way of saying that we can trust that what others (in this instance, a parent or caregiver) say is true, because in time and through experience, they have vali-dated our experience of the true nature of reality. They have been sympathetic to all the crucial things about us, and they have noticed and understood us for who we are, as we are. In the best scenario, there is a "communicative authenticity" that allows us to feel relaxed, at ease, and able to "interact with the world in predictable, trustwor-thy ways." As we grow, Dr. Siegel writes, "relationships that engender epistemic trust enable us to build a relational self that feels safe and a core inner self that feels whole and coherent. Coherence involves the experience of being connected." As we grow and mature, that trust and sense of self "unfolds" with people other than our parents, such as teachers, leaders, bosses, public figures, and more. But when this trust is broken, Dr. Siegel writes, things can go sideways. Our "survival" drives of anger, fear, and sadness—emotions that can work for us in good ways when we are well-regulated—can switch into over-drive and shift us from a "brain state of receptivity, with trust and safety, to one of reactivity, with mistrust and a sense of danger."

Also in on this important discussion is Dr. Gordon Neufeld, a world-renowned developmental psychologist with forty years of experience with children and youth and those responsible for them. A leading authority on child development, he's also the co-author, with Dr. Gabor Maté, of *Hold On to Your Kids*. Like Dr. Schore and Dr. Siegel, he believes nothing is more important for our emotional survival and ability to thrive than the quality of our first relationships. Everything, he told me, unfolds from there.

> **Dr. Gordon Neufeld:** Relationship is a context for everything. For parenting, for teaching, for raising the child. The interesting thing about the word *context* is that it's *con*, meaning "with," and *text*, referring to words. Like in a play, it's what comes with the words, but it's not the words. And because it's not the words, we're not conscious of it.
>
> **Sophie Grégoire:** So those roots that we don't see, where the unique beginning of our individual stories are found, would you call that the first bonds of attachment?
>
> **GN:** Yes, and if all goes well, these bonds continue to develop. The baby starts out seeking closeness through the senses— through smell, through hearing, through touch, through sight. But this quickly develops in toddlerhood to pursuing closeness through being the same as. In the third year this should expand to seeking closeness through belonging and loyalty. And if it's safe to unfold, the fourth year is all about mattering to those

you are attached to. If all goes well, the seeds of emotional intimacy are sown in the fifth year, often manifested by the child giving his or her heart to those the child is attached to. This is the point where the connection feels forever, answering the problems involved with the more superficial roots of attachment. Once the heart is given, the bias will be to share all that is within one's heart to those who have their hearts. This self-disclosure is the beginning of the capacity for psychological intimacy and sets the stage for lifelong growth.

So the physical bonds that form in the first year should continue to develop into deep roots of connection and relationship. The attachment of the baby is just the beginning of the story. Really, the brain is incredible in how it answers the most significant problem of life: how to hold when apart. Each of the ways of attaching answers inadequacies in the previous way of holding on. So when you can't be *with* [someone] all the time, at least you can be *like*. But if you can't be *like* all the time, because you're becoming different, at least you're part of, you *belong to*, and you're on the same side as. But if you can't be on the same side as all the time, or belonging, at least you *matter to*. But if you don't matter all the time—maybe because there's a new baby, or other things take priority from time to time—at least you've *given your heart to*. So you still have that emotional connection.

And then, finally, to share all that is within your heart. And this sets the stage for lifelong growth, and intimate relationships, and so on. The beginning is important, but so is the continuity of relationship. Because by the time you get to giving your heart to Mom and Dad, the beautiful thing about that is, that relationship is forever.

And so there we have it: the way our primary caregiver interacts with us in the two first years of life allows for our emotional attachment experiences to be regulated or dysregulated. For better or for worse, we are neurobiologically imprinted with secure or insecure attachments. What does that mean for us as adults? So much more than what we might imagine! While we certainly can't blame everything that happens in our adult lives on our childhood or the way we were parented, understanding more about these issues does help us gain a deeper sense of our own personality and all the ways our attachment style unconsciously expresses itself in our day-to-day lives.

As Allan Schore says: "Modern attachment theory is fundamentally more than safety and a secure base. It's about intimacy and connectedness." It also allows us to better understand and treat all sorts of attachment disorders, psychiatric symptoms, and personality disorders.

Obviously, no one feels fully secure at all times—nor is this the goal we seek. The aim is to develop the ability to detect the triggers that send our nervous systems into insecure places and learn how to come back to feeling secure, to be in tune with our inner child so we can become more well-adjusted, compassionate, curious, and resilient adults, ready to cope with the obstacles of life and thrive as best as we can.

I learned a lot about my own attachment style through therapy, asking my mother questions about her emotional state during and after pregnancy, and reading up on this crucial matter. I've also observed my insecurities and the ways in which I get triggered in my own relationships, as well as my capacity to repair and co-repair any "ruptures" that might surface. It made me realize that if we stay curious about ourselves and each other, we can heal along the way. I asked Allan if he thought that, on some level, we unconsciously serve as therapists to each other, and whether we need each other's actions and reactions to develop and thrive.

Dr. Allan Schore: To know ourselves is more than to know what our conscious minds are. Really, the key is that we have overlooked the importance of the unconscious mind. The right hemisphere [of the brain] is dominant for processing unconscious emotions. When we're in a situation where, all of a sudden, those strong emotions are out there, and we don't understand why, that's the point when we need to be able to listen to what our body is saying.

[Neuropsychiatrist] Iain McGilchrist has written about how, in today's Western culture, too much emphasis is placed on the left hemisphere and its drive for control, and less on the right hemisphere and its central role in affiliation and connection. We are too biased toward thinking over emotion, on what we should *do* rather than how we should *be* with people. In a secure attachment bond the baby's right hemisphere depends upon the emotional connection with the mother. The baby first learns how to be with the mother, and then how to be with and *get along* with people. Again, that is different than the left brain, which learns how to be independent, to be in control, and to *get ahead* of other people. Essentially, we need communication and balance between both hemispheres.

Sophie Grégoire: So, when we talk about self-knowledge in terms of "I think, therefore I am," the truth under all that is "I sense, I feel, therefore I am"?

AS: That's exactly right. In 1994, the discussion finally started to move from cognition, thinking, to emotion. Descartes was redefined as "I feel, therefore I am."

SG: Without wanting to sound too utopic, would you say that if we work at a very young age to set more healthy attachment bonds, we might be better able to adapt to change as human beings, and that this, in turn, might lead to less suffering on a global level?

AS: I think so. The ability to regulate stress, to play, and to give and receive love are ways we can cope with this suffering. Now more than ever, we need to come together and actively pursue and maintain our right-brain deep emotional connections with the people closest to us.

Getting to Know the Attachment Styles
WITH DR. JOHN GREY

Learning more about the four main attachment styles is a first step toward figuring out your own bond of attachment. As we've learned, the bond you formed with your parents or caregivers is a key feature in your emotional landscape. Below are descriptions of the four main attachment styles, based on information provided by Dr. John Grey, psychologist and author of *Five-Minute Relationship Repair* (we'll get to know Dr. Grey better in chapter 5). Note that these attachment styles are not mutually exclusive. You can engage with any of them at a particular time or moment, although one is usually dominant.

SECURE: Those of us with a secure attachment style had caregivers who tuned in to our emotional needs and responded consistently to our distress signals (like crying). They responded with support, using touch, holding, rocking, or a soothing voice. In such ways, they "co-regulated" us. As a result, we learned that we could count on our caregivers to respond when we were distressed. We felt safe and secure in their care, and probably soothed easily and settled down quickly.

INSECURE AVOIDANT: Those of us with an insecure avoidant attachment style had caregivers who didn't respond very much, if at all, to our emotional needs. When we signalled distress, they often ignored us, and co-regulatory responses such as supportive touch and holding were rarely used. As a result, we learned to self-soothe. We likely didn't cry very often and got good at entertaining ourselves. We learned to be self-sufficient and "low maintenance," often by suppressing our emotions.

INSECURE PREOCCUPIED (ALSO CALLED ANXIOUS-AMBIVALENT OR ANGRY RESISTANT): Those of us with an insecure preoccupied attachment style had caregivers who sometimes—but not consistently— responded to our distress signals with holding and supportive touch. Perhaps because of instability in the home or because our caregivers were sometimes unavailable, we were often left alone when distressed. We may also have dealt with role reversal, where we were expected to deal with caregivers or adults who were not well-regulated. As a result, we were often angry or hard to soothe; we could also be clingy and "high-maintenance."

DISORGANIZED: Those of us with this attachment style experienced danger or fear in our environment, perhaps due to a dysregulated caregiver. This presented us with an impossible dilemma: we needed our caregiver but, at the same time, were afraid of them and may even have needed to escape (in cases of physical or emotional abuse). The result was a highly dysregulated "push-pull" state. We pulled someone in to feel connected. We pushed them away to feel safe.

Where do you think you fit in? If you're not sure, there are many "find your attachment style" quizzes online. These shouldn't be substituted for a professional opinion, but they can help you self-screen before seeking advice.

A Happy Childhood?

Have you been reading this chapter and thinking, "I'm good. I'm safe, secure, regulated. My childhood was great"? If so, that's terrific. There's no doubt that those happy experiences have had a positive impact on your life. But I've also got some news for you: no matter how happy you think your childhood was, the truth is that we all carry some sort of trauma. I've learned this from the accomplished Dr. Gabor Maté, who has written several bestselling books, including *The Myth* of Normal, *In the Realm of Hungry Ghosts*, *Scattered Minds*, and *When the Body Says No*. He is also the co-author (with Dr. Gordon Neufeld) of *Hold On to Your Kids*. His works have been published internationally in more than thirty languages. Who better, really, to tackle this tough topic with us?

During our insightful chat, Dr. Maté explained how a "happy childhood" may not, in fact, be as happy or secure as we recall—and why that matters. Trauma comes in all shapes and sizes, and we carry even the smallest ones in our emotional baggage as we grow and attempt to relate to others in our world. I started by asking Dr. Maté to explain the difference between big-T and small-t traumas.

> **Dr. Gabor Maté:** The big-T traumas are linked to "outer shelter" experiences—sexual, physical, emotional abuse, neglect, a parent dying, a parent being mentally ill, a parent being addicted, violence in the family, a rancorous divorce. We can also add racism and poverty as social factors. War as well.
>
> The small-t traumas are not the bad things that happened, but the good things that should have happened but didn't. For example, having somebody to listen to you when you're sad. Being alone can ruin a child, even though nobody did anything bad to them. Because when you ask people, "When you were one day old, did you express your hurt or your upset?" the answer is of course they did. Have you ever met a one-day-old baby that doesn't express how they feel? So something happened between one day and three years, say, where you learned that you had to keep it to yourself. That's a small-t trauma.
>
> **Sophie Grégoire:** And how does this influence our capacity for regulation?
>
> **GM:** Well, there are two kinds of regulation. Self-suppression is a regulation. You have anger or sadness, but you repress it, so you don't even feel it. Well, now you've regulated it, but it's a self-damaging regulation, which has all kinds of consequences later on in physical and mental health. Then there's regulation

when you're experiencing the emotion, but you're able to actually regulate how you deal with it, so that's a freedom, that's consciousness.

So I say there's the pseudo-regulation, which is repression, and then there's the genuine regulation, which is being aware—fully aware—of one's emotions and then choosing how to deal with them. And that has to develop over time; that's a function of maturation, and that maturation can only take place if there are adults around who are nurturing you and who are self-regulated themselves.

SG: Some people reading this might be thinking, "Wow, this is all really interesting, but it doesn't apply to me. I'm secure. I had a good childhood. I'm not traumatized at all." Do you hear that in your work?

GM: Absolutely. But most people who say that are just not aware of their trauma. Because some people's definition of *trauma* is, you know, the very terrible things that happen—like the residential schools, like genocide, like all the abuse that some people experience—and they don't realize that *trauma* means "a wound," and people can be wounded, even if they weren't horribly mistreated. There are many ways to wound human beings. It takes me three minutes, usually, to actually get underneath that.

SG: What is it that you ask people?

GM: I usually ask them about their childhood experience. You've actually looked at your trauma, Sophie, but let's say you hadn't. If I'd asked you, "What was your childhood like?" would you have said, "I had a happy childhood"?

SG: Yes, I would say so, mostly, yes.

GM: Then I would have asked you, "Was there any yelling in your house?"

SG: Yes, sometimes.

GM: Then I would ask you, "How old were you when you heard the yelling?"

SG: Very young.

GM: Then I would have asked you, "How did you feel when you heard the yelling?"

SG: Sad, fearful. Actually, I remember counting the flowers on the wall-covering in my bedroom to divert my attention when I would hear my parents argue.

GM: Then I would have asked you, "Who did you speak to about your sadness?"

SG: No one, I guess. I was an only child.

GM: Okay. Then I would have asked you, "Do you have children?"

SG: Yes.

GM: Then I would have asked you, "If they were three years old and they felt sad, who would you want them to speak to?"

SG: Me.

GM: Then I would have asked you, "If you found out that your three-year-old was sad and she didn't tell you about it, how would you explain that?"

SG: That they didn't feel safe to tell me.

GM: What's it like for a three-year-old not to feel safe?

SG: Awful.

GM: There's your happy childhood.

SG: Wow. Okay. What if someone tells you that they know and remember what happened to them as a child, but that is the past and it's behind them?

GM: If it's true, that's wonderful, but I want to see how they're functioning. This is just an example, but let's say your partner doesn't want to sleep with you, and right away, you perceive that you're rejected and you're hurt—then your childhood is not behind you. Because all that happened was that your partner said, "Not tonight," and there could be any number of reasons why they said that. But if you go right away to "I'm hurt, rejected, abandoned"—or any kind of painful emotions—then your childhood is not behind you.

If somebody calls you stupid and you get all upset, your

childhood is not behind you. Because to an adult, what does it matter what somebody else says? But if you're dependent on other people's opinion, then you're still a child.

So, [when] people say, "My childhood is behind me," I want to see what their lives are like, how they relate to themselves, to their work, to their relationships, to their children. That's where we find out if your childhood is really behind you.

SG: Have you drawn links between childhood trauma and personality and afflictions in adulthood?

GM: All these dynamics, whether avoidant or disorganized or whatever, are just designed to protect the child. And all the personality traits that people develop, that I write about as being the emotional templates for physical illness—for example, being super-nice, being super-accommodating, super-compliant, repressing anger, being helpful to everybody—they have the *effect* of being self-sabotaging, but they don't have the *intention* of being self-sabotaging. There's no intention to ruin anything. In fact, there's an intention to preserve something.

SG: As an only child, I can still sense somewhere inside me that I was trying to preserve my relationship with my parents as the central axis of my life. The little Sophie wanted to make everything okay for her parents. Does that make sense?

GM: Yes. The intention is to protect something, which is the relationship. And the child is desperately dependent on that relationship, but when the child complies and tries to please the adult to make things work, and ignores their own needs, that ends up hurting and stressing the child.

SG: What is emotional maturity to you?

GM: It's being in the present moment, knowing what my needs are, not confusing my needs with my desires. Knowing what my emotions are and being able to choose how I can express them. So, in other words, being an adult person in the present moment, in touch with myself and not confusing the present with the past.

37

SG: What's the biggest lesson you've learned from all the patients you've seen, from all the trauma you've witnessed and helped heal along the way?

GM: It's that most people are unconscious—in other words, they're not aware—of what moves them. And that liberation is possible. If you're not conscious of something, you can hardly be responsible for it. In that sense, there are very few responsible people.

Dr. Maté always provides such food for thought. I hope you've learned some things about your bond of attachment or the big-T or little-t traumas that were part of your childhood. But no matter what this conversation has brought to light, it's important to know that these patterns are not stuck in stone. They can change over the course of our lives. It all depends on the awareness and care we bring to ourselves, our experiences, the people we surround ourselves with, and our habits. Dr. Siegel uses a term that speaks intensely to me: *becoming whole*. In order to become whole, and to take our best selves out into the wider world and approach others from a place of trust, it is paramount that we understand our own tendencies, learn together, and acknowledge ruptures and make repairs as our life unfolds. This demands presence, deep listening, and collaboration. And the sooner we start—with ourselves and with the young people in our lives—the better.

Now, as a mother of two teenagers, I know first-hand how taxing it can be to encourage our children to be present and collaborative, to be deep listeners. Once they hit those early teen years, they are determined to find their own identity, separate from us—which is how it should be. But they are also doing it in a culture that is obsessed with the "self," and that presents distractions at every turn. We can encourage them to block out the noise and take time to explore their emotional landscape, to listen to what their deepest thoughts and feelings are telling them, but they may not always listen to us—at least in the moment. Whether we're parenting teens ourselves, teaching or coaching them, or interacting with these wonderfully complex humans in another way, it's important to know what they are dealing with as they navigate the turbulent waters of the teenage years, and to prepare ourselves to support them through whatever comes their way.

So let's dive into these agitated waters. Whether you're parenting one or more teens, or just recalling your own quiet or explosive rebellion, this next chapter is for all of us.

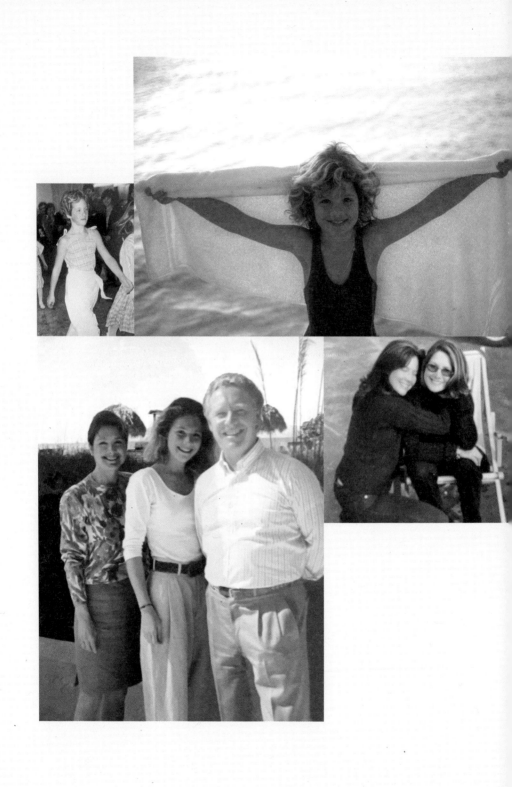

2

Growing Up

The Teen in All of Us

The passage from childhood to independence is a rough and winding road,
with potholes, bumps, and hollows, like a country lane after a spring thaw.

ARLENE STAFFORD-WILSON

Is there an image of yourself that comes to mind when you remember your teenage years? What does it look like? You can think about these questions no matter your age—even if you're still in your teenage years, or not terribly far removed. What sense or memory do you have of your own time and space? Time enjoyed with friends or family? A special moment with a love interest, or a huge fight with your parents? It's interesting to realize what we carry with us from certain stages of our life. What instantly comes to mind for me are my love interests and my after-school routine. I remember snapshots of that as if it were yesterday. It sometimes went like this:

41

- Jump on the city bus for the ride to my neighbourhood, and then walk home from the bus stop.
- Ring the doorbell and wait for my mother to answer. (I had a key, but most of the time, I knew she was there and liked the ritual of waiting for her to let me in.)
- Put my school bag down, wiggle out of my blouse, and toss my bra to the floor; change out of my uniform.
- Throw an occasional fit for no specific reason. (I would roll around on the carpet whining about something or other, which led my mother to call these episodes "carpet crises." My daughter now has her own version of the "carpet crisis." I let her have it, but I make sure we find something to share and laugh about together afterwards.)
- Have one snack and then another, because I'm famished. (I was a growing girl, after all.)
- Head up to my room, play the *Family Feud* game on my huge IBM computer (yes, the one with the black screen and green letters). Maybe look at myself in the mirror and sing, or look at myself from all angles, making model faces. Criticize something about my appearance while comparing myself to my favourite singer (who had more muscles and a stage) or my favourite actress (who had longer legs and a smaller nose). So much time wasted in front of mirrors, I tell you!
- Study and talk on the phone (for way too long) with a friend or a boy I had a crush on.
- Eat dinner early, most often by myself in front of the television, while watching *The Oprah Winfrey Show*, *The Golden Girls*, *Three's Company*, *The Facts of Life*, *The Cosby Show*, *The Fresh Prince of Bel-Air*, *A Different World*—the list goes on. (Apart from on the occasional Sunday evening, we didn't eat together as a family, and when we did, it rarely went well. Things would start on a good note, but soon enough, my father would be dismissive with my mom or act like a complete recluse, and I would feel hurt, sad, and angry.)

Does any of this sound familiar? It's funny how these days, as a mother of two teenagers, I see some similarities between my typical after-school behaviours and theirs. I can relate to many parents (and teenagers themselves) who find navigating this tumultuous period of life challenging. Don't get me wrong: I adore my two teens and am deeply proud of them—both for who they are now and who they are becoming—

Cry. Forgive.

Learn. Move on.

Let your tears water

the seeds of your

future happiness.

STEVE MARABOLI

but I could definitely take less of the sassiness, mood swings, eye-rolling, criticizing, questionable risk-taking, and other hallmarks of this age. I know very well, though, that it's all part of growing up, and I feel so privileged to accompany them on this path. I also know I'm far from the only one trying my best to guide my teens while also giving them some leeway to figure out their own stuff.

I've been working with and listening to young people for two decades now through my advocacy work, and I've come to know that teenagers are beautifully sensitive beings who are trying to make sense of themselves and of the world. This is not an easy task. The pressures they live with today are similar to some of the struggles my generation went through, but the cultural, environmental, and socio-economic factors have changed. The planet was troubled then and it still is troubled—that's the bad news. The good news is that it is also filled with incredible young humans whose level of awareness is allowing them to see the world as it is and face the truth about the challenges ahead, both for the planet and in their own lives. When we face the truth, we can find solutions to every problem. Today's teens and young people are also so much more in tune with their mental well-being than we ever were. That doesn't mean life is easier for them than it was for us—far from it—but we, as a society, have finally started to talk more about the importance of mental health in our daily lives, and that's a huge step forward.

Walking a New Path

In chapter 1, we talked about how childhood is where everything starts, where our emotional and neurological patterns begin to form and imprint on the brain. But as hormones kick in and we seek more independence, we walk a new path of self-discovery, attempting to defy the norms and affirm ourselves. If we feel safe enough, we know we can embark on this journey without losing the love of our family. We enter a phase where the transformations in our brain are as intense as the changes in our bodies.

I'd like to share more of the conversation I had with the brilliant Dr. Gordon Neufeld, whom we met in chapter 1. Gordon's own children have given him six grandchildren, whom he still cares for and learns from. His wisdom is equal to his tenderness: "We must remember that we are all hungry to exist in somebody else's presence," he told me. "I'm seventy-five and I still have that need. We all do." Here, he shares some fascinating insights on the transition between childhood and the teenage years.

Sophie Grégoire: What are some of the biggest challenges that our young people face as they move out of childhood and into their teens?

Dr. Gordon Neufeld: The difficulty for today's adolescents is when closeness and selfhood are different paths. When becoming a separate being is at the cost of closeness and attachment to parents, we have a problem, because they're in a dreadful conflict.

In adolescence, they face a lot of separation of all kinds, and for all kinds of reasons, it's going to be very difficult to feel as if Mom and Dad are holding on to them. Or as if they can hold on to Mom and Dad. And so the deeper the attachment—if they're attached at the heart, by sharing, and by not having any secrets that divide—the more they are able to be their own person without it being at the cost of being close.

The most important thing ever as parents is to give two invitations: the invitation to exist in my presence and for that to be unconditional, and the invitation to experience the fruit of that—to become one's own person. The adolescent is fortunate when both things can be true simultaneously. "I can be close to Mom and Dad, and be my own person at the same time." That saves them from a huge conflict that is unnecessary in adolescence.

We've been thinking of adolescence in far too superficial a way. We think they need to separate to grow up. Does a plant need to separate to grow up? Oh my goodness, no. It needs to be deeper rooted to grow up. So we've been making a fundamental mistake in our thinking.

SG: How do we help teenagers who struggle because they didn't and don't have a healthy attachment bond?

GN: We focus on the attachment. You don't pull a plant up by the roots. Our job is to support, to nurture the relationships. To convey to the adolescent that I will hold on to you no matter what. Through thick and thin, whatever comes. You can depend upon that. And if that message gets through, then the teenager, the brain, is free to go to the other agenda, which is to think for myself. To make my own decisions. But as soon as the attachment is in question, then all the energy goes to attachment again.

Now, the problem in our society is that children reattach to their peers and that looks like independence, but that's not independence. That's transferred dependence. That's not independence at all.

SG: So teenagers have to feel safe before they go out and explore?

GN: Yes, to feel safe in the contact and closeness with those who care for them. A parent, a grandma, an aunt. There just has to be somebody to whom they are strongly attached that says, "I've got you. I am holding on to you. Nothing is going to come between you and me." Something that is able to convey a resting place.

SG: We've been treating the teenage years as an age of rebellion. Is it really a rebellion?

GN: We're calling a lot of things rebellion. And we're all allergic to coercion. We don't like to be told what to do and be pushed around. That is a universal instinct. It was a psychoanalyst over one hundred years ago who called it "counter-will," and I think that's a beautiful name for it. If you resist the will that's imposed upon you.

Now, we have idealized that in adolescence. Counter-will is meant to protect a child from being bossed around by anybody they're not attached to. So, if their neighbour tells them what to do, then they say, "No, you can't tell me what to do. You're not my mommy." Which is exactly the point.

SG: Yeah, but they'll tell the mommy, "Hey, Mommy, you can't tell me what to do. I'm fourteen now." What mistake, from a communication point of view, do parents make when we address our teenagers?

GN: If you tell your partner what to do, they'll balk. Unless, first of all, you've got a connection. We forget this with our teenagers. They need contact and closeness. When you come alongside of them, when you get a connection, when you can get some nods and smiles, you've got a context in which to be able to discuss things, in which to be able to give direction, to give guidance. I call it "collecting." That's why you start the dance with their eyes—getting a smile, getting a nod or two. And then you can go to work.

But we parent cold. We must not parent cold. That is the mistake we make with our adolescents. We think it's about their thinking. It's not. We have to have their hearts to be able to have a context for our teaching, for our parenting.

SG: Can we talk about the importance of physical presence, one nervous system in front of another nervous system? Sometimes teenagers don't want to be touched. How do we deal with that?

GN: Well, it's a dance. It's a courtship, you know? If the eyes don't come easily, say something. Work for the ears—something that will give them a smile, that will warm them up, that will get a nod.

We just have to be patient with the beginning. We're so much in a hurry. We don't create the context. At least with our babies, we know we have to connect, connect, connect, and connect. But we forget this—that we are creatures of attachment for life. It isn't over ever. Ever. Our wounds are in attachment. It doesn't matter how individuated one is. And when we don't get it from the people who are important to us, we're stung. We're wounded.

SG: I have chills. You've made me realize that we move much too quickly with teenagers. The rhythm of love is slow. And we slow down for babies, but do we slow down for teenagers?

GN: Yes, that's exactly it, Sophie, exactly yes. We don't start at the beginning, you see? We take things for granted. And we can't take them for granted. We are hungry for this invitation to exist in another's presence. An adolescent is hungry, and if they aren't feeding at our table, they'll be feeding at somebody else's table. And that won't necessarily be in their best interests.

SG: What happens in the brains of teenagers that makes their moods go up and down, and makes them become more irritable? Is it a biological predisposition, or is this also something that we've branded so much that it's almost like a cultural contagion?

GN: It's both, really. It is developmental. That is, the pubescent, the post-pubescent, is facing more separation in their life. More physical separation, emotional separation, separation of all kinds in their attachments. And that's both developmental and it's societal. And unfortunately, too many parents are throwing in the towel. They don't realize that this cascading care is meant for life.

Now, what happens when adolescents face more separation is, as we know now, it evokes primal emotions. It evokes frustration, it evokes alarm, intensified pursuit. These are

CLOSER TOGETHER

47

powerful, powerful emotions. Never mind all the hormonal changes from becoming a sexual being capable of procreating.

The finishing touch of all maturation is basically to be able to feel conflicted—part of me feels this way, thinks this way, and part of me feels that. However, when a young adolescent is over-whelmed, they go back to the preschooler stage of exhibiting all of the signs of being on a pendulum swing. Because when emotions are large, we can't feel them at the same time. And so the child is frustrated, and then in intense pursuit, and then in intense alarm.

SG: How does a parent help modulate those emotions?

GN: Well, making room for them is best. There's way too much emphasis on trying to control emotion instead of making space for emotion. One of the biggest mistakes we've made is the construct of self-regulation. Because what they need is space. Space to feel. They need safe relationships to feel. The research is unequivocal this way.

The adolescent needs stories, and music, and art, and paint-ing, and dance, and more. Not to become better than others, just as emotional playgrounds. We are so busy trying to get children to get a hold of themself, control themself, regulate themself, that we're forgetting something far more important: the more space we give an emotion to exist, and the more we can get it to where it's playful rather than free of repercussions, the less room it takes. And the secret to self-control is mixed feelings.

Talking with Gordon about self-regulation reminded me of some-thing I'd read. In her book *Dopamine Nation: Finding Balance in the Age of Indulgence*, Dr. Anna Lembke, professor of psychiatry at Stanford University School of Medicine, asks, "Why, in a time of unprecedented wealth, freedom, technological progress, and medical advancement, do we appear to be unhappier and in more pain than ever?" Her answer? "The reason why we're miserable may be because we're working so hard to avoid being miserable."

Dr. Lembke explains that our brain processes pain and pleasure in the same spot, and the neuro-relationship between the two is something like the tipping point in the movement of a see-saw. The trick isn't to avoid one and embrace the other, but to allow ourselves to experience it all and find balance. This can be messy—especially in the teenage years, when emotions are all over the place—but it's so necessary. I shared this idea with Gordon as we continued our conversation:

SG: So, basically, emotions need the space to exist in order to be lived fully and to dissipate? In a way, the heart's unfinished or unfelt business ends up cluttering our minds?

GN: Yeah. Emotion, as we know now, has purpose. Alarm is meant to move us to caution. Frustration is meant to move us to change things. Intense pursuit is meant to close the gap. Every emotion has purpose.

Emotions have to be felt for the work to be finished. When you feel an emotion, now you are capable of feeling mixed feelings. You can feel the futility. Then it makes you sad. Which means that you know something cannot work, will not work. Emotions have to be felt for the work to be finished. And that needs space, and room. And so the most important thing is to feel it, not control it.

SG: Why are teenagers so anxious these days? What's happening with their brains?

GN: First of all, the emotional root of anxiety is alarm. The universal trigger for alarm in the brain is facing separation. So, if we ask the question "Why the anxiety?" it's because of facing separation. The problem is that anxiety has to do with an idea of the alarm displaced.

SG: According to the dictionary, the amygdala is a roughly almond-shaped mass of grey matter inside each cerebral hemisphere, involved with the experiencing of emotions. It also detects threat and activates the appropriate fear-related

49

behaviours in response to threat. Is our culture activating the amygdala more than it was, say, two hundred years ago?

GN: Well, the nuclear family is the smallest it's ever been. Children used to be in a context of a village of attachment, where there was some kind of permanence of connection. We send our children out from the home to be raised, but we don't create the context that is required first of all. Children are meant to be raised by those they're attached to. So their alarm is all over the place.

And so, yes, that is true for all of society, but what is the answer? We're facing overwhelming separation, and the language needs to change. We've gone way too far with this anxiety bit, and way too far pathologizing it. If we would only get back to all of the earlier understandings, [which are] that it's all about facing separation. What's normal is that we all want closeness so badly.

When there is no rest from anxiety, when one is anxiety-ridden, it tells me that the person, the child, whoever they are, has not yet had their tears of sadness—the feelings of futility, the sadness about the things they could not change in their life.

SG: I love to listen to sad music, and I see my teenage daughter and her friends enjoying it, too. Is that typical behaviour?

GN: That is a really healthy response. You see, music can make sadness sweet. It's the only thing, really, that can make sadness sweet enough to bear sometimes. You make room and space for the feelings to take care of you, and they'll take care of us.

SG: Going back to what we were discussing earlier about needing to fully experience our emotions, is sadness necessary and healthy for the teenager or young adult not just to feel but also for the development of a sense of passion and purpose?

GN: Absolutely! Absolutely! Sadness is saying, "Oh, something has to end before something else can begin." Your brain is on a track that isn't going to work. It's the brain registering that "Okay, we're walking a maze. We're at a blind alley here. There has to be a little death before there's more life."

There are no more melancholy periods in life than adolescence and old age. When I was on a sabbatical in Provence in '98 and '99, it was so interesting. Because at a fountain in the middle of the village were the grandparents and the adolescents. And it always struck me that, in many ways, they were at the same stage.

Adolescents can't hang on to childhood, right? And, of course, the elderly, they can't hold on to life as it is. There are so many things that they need to let go of. Like happiness lies on the other side of sadness that has not yet been felt.

SG: Is this distance we've created culturally between teenagers and the elderly because we're obsessed with youth? Because we do not accept our own mortality?

GN: Yes.

SG: And how is that affecting our brain health?

GN: Hugely, hugely. Earlier, I worked almost completely with Indigenous youth who were incarcerated. And the remarkable stories of recovery that I heard were almost always between an elder or a grandparent and a grandchild. And it was because in both cases, there's too much to bear. But they need the context of each other and the support to be able to do this. Parents are too busy to notice at this time in their lives, you know? And so the adolescents need their grandparents, and the grandparents need their adolescents.

The grandparents are generally saying, "Well, you know, do you have time? I made some fresh cookies for you. Do you have time?" And it's exactly what the adolescent needs.

Time and Temptations

Time is precious, isn't it? I don't think we realize that as we enter the teenage years. My friends and I sometimes felt as if we had all the time in the world, and that even wasting it wasn't a waste, because

51

there would always be more. There is something beautiful about that. Naive, of course, but maybe the carelessness of feeling that our lives might go on forever is necessary in order for our teenage selves to build dreams with the confidence that nothing will stop us along the way. Temptations arise at every step, and learning to navigate those demands discernment, even as we find ourselves in the heart of so many new experiences. As we begin to figure out what does or doesn't work for us, and to spread our wings and reach for independence, the road can feel bumpy indeed, marked by rises and falls.

I've definitely had a taste of both. As we learned with Gordon Neufeld, there is a biological need for the spaciousness of time, time to explore the vast fields inside ourselves and those that extend out into the world. Learning how to process conflicting emotions during the peak of hormonal changes is quite a balancing act. But feeling out of balance can act as a trigger, nudging us to use our inner compass to guide us toward what makes us feel whole, centred, and grounded.

For some of us, family can be part of that grounding—but family can also come with complications. I loved my family so much, and a big part of me wanted nothing more than to save my parents from them-selves and each other. As it had when I was younger, this feeling weighed on me throughout my teens. I felt like I shared my life with my mother more than with my dad. I also felt that my mom shared her life more with me than she did with her husband. I never saw them engag-ing in an activity together just for the sake of it. They spoke about playing doubles in tennis together when I was younger, and would joke about the fact that one time my mom hit my dad in the back of the head with the ball and that was the end of it. When he came home from work, he would spend time in the garden alone and then head straight into a little studio beside my bedroom, where he ate by himself.

Apart from living in the same house, my dad and I didn't really interact on a daily basis as I began stepping out of childhood. He would occasionally give me a lift to high school, although he preferred to listen to his favourite classical music station rather than talk to me. A quick "I love you. Have a good one," was exchanged at the drop-off, and that was about it. I have no recollection of discussing school, projects, friends, or anything about my teenage life with him apart from when the occasional crisis hit. And even then, the interaction was short and quick, and I was left feeling as if my mom had told him, "Go see Sophie. She's hurting badly. She needs you." Did I ever. He was there, in my home, but he wasn't. Not really.

I wanted to be perfect so my parents didn't need to worry about me—it seemed like they had enough to worry about between themselves. I wanted to save my mother from her own insecurities and save my dad from his relationship with himself. I guess that was a lot to carry. I didn't know then that we can sustain quality relationships only according to our own level of self-awareness. But I thought my strong shoulders and big heart could bear the weight.

Overall, my teenage life looked good from the outside, which only deepened my guilt over not being the perfect girl. Luckily, this didn't prevent me from experiencing joy, love, and other positive emotions. Outside of the challenges at home, I was what you might call a pretty typical teen. I enjoyed attending my all-girls school and was a curious student. I was quite disciplined and did my homework without the help of my parents. I loved keeping my notes clean and colourful, which meant that I was asked to lend them to friends on occasion. Succeeding in school was important to me, and I studied hard. Apart from math, I knew I could learn anything easily. I found something interesting in at least part of every subject matter, but I really loved gym. I had a visceral thirst to move. I wanted to explore the world without being supervised. I wanted to push my boundaries, both physically and mentally, without my parents having to worry about me. I wanted to taste life on my own without having to share an account of it. I wanted freedom, inside and out. Being athletic saved me in so many ways. It gave me a sense of independence and strength. Being adventurous and active was one of the ways I could test the playful and courageous warrior inside me.

One year, I tried out for the volleyball team. I liked the sport and was a good player, though not a great one, and I thrived on the competitive aspect of the game. I remember attending a tournament at another school in the province, where we slept in the gymnasium and ate from vending machines. I wanted to taste everything in there, from the submarine sandwiches to the potato chips and chocolate bars. I somehow knew not to let my classmates see me overeat. Nothing was quite clear to me then when it came to my struggles with food; it was all tied up with self-esteem, control over my life and my own body, and so much more. I could feel that something was off within myself, but I thought it would pass.

As most teenagers do, I loved going out with my friends to parties, but I was never a big drinker. Usually, I was the first one to start the party (early) and the first one to leave (also early). I had seen so many people drink too much—to the point of getting really sick, and even to unconsciousness. It wasn't pretty, and I never felt as if I needed lots of booze to either have fun or numb my emotions. I didn't think of it this way at the time, but I guess I had enough numbing going on with my growing addiction to food. I also came from a family where I saw overdrinking lead to problems, so that knowledge was always in the back of my mind. Plus, I never wanted to waste the early part of the next day recovering from a hangover when I could get up early and start moving instead.

Although I was quite social, I was also a loner at times. I had two or three close girlfriends, and we always had fun together, but sometimes at lunch, I would decide to head off on a walk by myself. I was very aware of the gossip, jealousy, and peer pressure that could creep into relationships at this age. I think it's possible that I kept my friend groups fairly small to avoid competition and rejection. I never enjoyed arguing with my girlfriends and always tried to speak openly about tensions. I also really enjoyed hanging out with boys, mostly because of their intrepid nature, their sense of humour, and how they loved pulling pranks with me. While I felt at home with them, I was also keenly aware of being observed. I wanted them to like me, to treat me like one of them. I also wanted to be their favourite girl. It was a space of growth and camaraderie, but also a space of trying to please, to feel loved.

Thinking about those mixed-up feelings now, I realize that I was quite aware, even then, of the feminine and masculine energy dancing inside of me. I loved to lead and be led, care and be cared for, fight and be fought for. I am as tender as I am forceful, as quiet as I am wild. I've since learned not to shy away from these aspects of my personality but to foster them in different ways. Looking back, I can see that I was craving to be the truest, most balanced version of myself. I just needed more life experience to turn that craving into a reality.

I've also learned to look at my relationships with boys during that time through the lens of my changing relationship with my father. Like so many teen girls, I was in love with being in love. I would sit in class and stare at my boyfriend's picture, just daydreaming away. I'd look at his turquoise eyes, his dark, curly hair, his charming dimpled smile (I guess I have a type), and practise signing my first name beside his last name, just to see how it looked and sounded. Ugh. I know: it's clear to me now that I was probably trying to fill the gap left by my dad's emotional absence by reaching for male emotional presence and connection in other ways. I knew my dad loved me, but he was no longer emotionally present in my day-to-day life. I internalized that sense of abandonment and the sadness that came with it.

When I was about fourteen, I attended a tennis camp near Mont-Tremblant. I had taken tennis lessons prior to camp and loved the sport. I had some basic talent, just like my dad did, but I also had much to learn. On the day I arrived, there were a couple of very cute male campers dressed in tennis clothes sitting near the drop-off area. My smile stretched from ear to ear as I waved goodbye to my parents. (My mom later shared with me the thought that was running through her head as they drove away: "Oh my, what have we done?")

I certainly put a lot of work into my tennis game that summer and improved in many areas, but there were plenty of distractions, too—mostly of the "boy" variety. There was Hunter from Boston, who was kind and caring. I think I kissed him, but I mostly remember being out on the lake with him and having him confide, "I wish life was one long afternoon in a canoe." Sigh. But I had a more serious crush on a certain gorgeous counsellor. He was too old for me (at least nineteen, maybe even in his early twenties), but he gave me just enough attention to feed the story I was writing for us in my head. I don't know what I was *thinking* (probably something subconscious about a connection with an older male), but my body sure knew what it was *feeling*. We were all walking along the road one day when he told me he was attracted to me and felt like he was a lion and I was a kitten. I would run far away if I heard that today, but back then, I was curious to explore, to get his full attention.

Apart from one kiss—before which he asked me, "Are you ready?" to which my fourteen-year-old self answered, "No ... are *you* ready?"— nothing ever happened between me and the older counsellor. He lived not far away from me, and after I got home from camp, I rode past his place on my bike way too many times that summer.

There was one counsellor at the camp whose energy repulsed me. He was a bit older than most of the staff and quite denigrating to one of the female coaches, Colleen, whom I loved. Once, he hung her dirty underwear on the cafeteria wall for everyone to see. I was in shock—as were many of the other campers. That same week, he was playing games with campers and told us we needed to find a quick team chant. He told us he would shout, "Cindy's in the bush," and instructed us to reply, "Rape!"

Writing this now makes me feel sick. I was so young then, too young to even consider reporting him to the camp director. Although most of the campers (especially the female ones) thought the counsellor was a creep, and even some of the guys had our backs, this was not a time when you could denounce someone in a position of authority for such a "silly thing" as the toxic vibe we got from him. But for me, and many other young women, he was the embodiment of a certain type of angry, repressed, and misogynistic man—the kind that made me feel as if girls and women simply weren't as safe as boys were when it came to roaming and exploring our world. Danger was always lurking around some corner.

56

This episode reminds me of others where I was forced to confront how vulnerable young women can be. One of my closest friends developed a friendship with our history teacher, who must have been in his sixties. At first, we all celebrated their fun and knowledge-sharing bond, but it ended up in a room with a door he locked, and my girlfriend felt completely uneasy and asked to leave. Thank goodness for the #MeToo movement and the wave of truth-telling it has unleashed. This doesn't mean situations like these don't happen anymore, but it does mean that it's harder for them to go unnoticed. When people tell their story, it allows for others to do the same. There is power in that.

My own brush with toxic masculinity (I've come to believe that all women have had at least one) came around the same time. It was late afternoon and I was on the city bus, making my way home from high school. The ride took about half an hour, and I was sitting by myself in the middle of the bus. At the back were a couple of teenage boys being a bit rambunctious. I could hear their voices and see them out of the corner of my eye. A couple of minutes later, the boys started making comments about my big hair. Then I heard them talking about my lips: "Looks like you got a pair that can suck!" With my heart pounding in my chest, I moved to the bench right beside the driver. I didn't want to ask for his help, though, as I was scared it would make things worse. That ride seemed eternal. The part when I finally got off the bus is blurry in my memory, but I do recall one of those boys touching my hair as he exited the bus after me. I was about a hundred metres away from home and started running for my life. I never looked back. For many months, I was often nervous while taking the bus, but fortunately, I didn't see those boys again. I was lucky it ended the way it did. Women and girls across the world experience this fear on a daily basis, in situations where their physical and emotional safety have been compromised. Living in fear is not living. In many ways, it's simply surviving.

The Big Five: The Neurochemicals behind Most Teen Behaviour

WITH DR. SHIMI KANG

When it comes to parenting teens in this overstimulating world, Dr. Shimi Kang is an expert. She's an award-winning psychiatrist and community activist, and the bestselling author of *The Dolphin Parent* and *The Tech Solution: Creating Healthy Habits for Kids Growing Up in a Digital World*. In *The Tech Solution*, she identifies "five key neurochemicals that regulate your children's lives, making them feel energetic or unmotivated, connected or lonely, happy or unhappy, engaged or withdrawn from life. Dopamine, cortisol, endorphin, oxytocin, and serotonin are often referred to as the body's 'chemical messengers.'" As Dr. Kang writes, "They exist in every human, and trigger responses that are as certain as the rising of the sun. And by understanding them, we can help our kids learn to fire and wire healthy habits that will leave them feeling content, valued, empowered, loved."

As you read the descriptions below (adapted from the book), try to imagine what it might feel like if these neurochemicals were way out of balance. What might the consequences be for our bodies, minds, and society if the very building blocks of human health were targeted, manipulated, and dysregulated?

1. **Dopamine** drives our motivation, rewarding us with an immediate sense of pleasure. It's mainly released by activities that promote species survival, such as hunting, gathering, and sexual activity. Since we are no longer living as our prehistoric ancestors did, our modern-day "hunting" might be levelling up in a video game. "Gathering" might be collecting social media likes.

2. **Cortisol** and the stress response produce feelings of being under attack. When dangers arise, cortisol and the stress response urge us to do something to escape—whether it is freeze, fight, or flight. This causes our heart rate and blood pressure to spike. Over time, this can lead to sleep impairment, weight gain, intestinal problems, and the suppression of the immune system; it can also interrupt the formation of bones.

3. **Endorphins** produce feelings of peace, calm, bliss, or euphoria and are released through activities like cardiovascular exercise, laughter, and sex. All of these counteract feelings of anxiety, stress, and pain. Endorphins provide relief from life's hardships, freeing us to innovate and try new things.

4. **Oxytocin** produces feelings of being safe and loved. It motivates us to trust and help others, seek companionship, and learn to love.

5. **Serotonin** produces feelings of contentment, happiness, pride, and respect. It motivates us to try new things, innovate, and gain respect from others.

Dr. Kang tells us that while young brains are wired and rewarded for risk-taking, novelty-seeking, peer admiration, and social connection, the frontal lobe—known as the brain's "control centre," and responsible for long-term thinking and an awareness of consequences—matures in the early to mid-twenties. It's a recipe for confusion, conflict, and even mental, physical, and social health challenges. As well, the dizzying pace of new social media trends, consumerism, and general global change make it next to impossible to provide teens with timely advice on every issue. Which is exactly why it's so important for our young people to know their own brains, and their power.

The Dangers of Too Much, Too Fast

I can't believe the roller coaster of emotions I let myself ride that summer at camp. It was all part of growing up—I know that now—but it makes me wonder what experiences and people my kids will encounter in their upcoming summers and years. I read once that it's better to inform our kids about and expose them to life in all its light and darkness than to shield them from it. How else will they prepare for their own adventures? Shelter them too much and at the first sign of something new, or tempting, or unexpected, they're likely to feel as if we've dropped them in the middle of Times Square on a busy Saturday night. Not sure about you, but I go into total sensory overload when I visit that place, and I can't stay for too long.

It's an evocative and useful metaphor when it comes to the tumultuous teen years—especially in this era when many of us have 24/7 access to technology and social media. Social media has transformed our lives, and our brains, for that matter, in ways we never could have anticipated, affecting everything from how we shop and play to how we communicate and interact with each other. Talk about sensory overload!

Dr. Lembke explores this modern, culture-specific sensory overload in *Dopamine Nation*. Just think about the "sensory inputs" teens face on a daily basis: flirting and sexting, drugs and alcohol, gambling and gaming, shopping and social media, and the list goes on. The available sources of intensely rewarding stimuli are everywhere. Dr. Lembke explains that each of these inputs sends a wave of dopamine to our brains, and that we can get addicted to that "feel good" boost. Teenagers, especially, seek these high-intensity sensory experiences, but too much pleasure can lead to pain. We all have to get better at embracing pain, at sitting with it and learning what it's trying to teach us. But we also have to be more aware of what this constant exposure to technology is doing to our brains at every age, especially with young people.

Dr. Mari Swingle is a practising clinician, researcher, and author of *i-Minds*. She has heard the stories of hundreds of children, teenagers, and their parents in her office over the years and has noticed some interesting trends.

Sophie Grégoire: In your practice, what changes have you noticed in children's brains and behaviours over the past two decades?

Dr. Mari Swingle: Well, if you've read my work, you know the answer that's coming: developmental changes associated with the overuse of interactive screen-based technology. I want to preface this by saying there's absolutely nothing wrong with a little use, if it's a complement. If kids kick a ball together, ride their bikes together, bug their siblings together, and then game or goof around on screens a bit together—that's modern childhood. But that's not what we're seeing. We're seeing interactive screen technologies used because children no longer have curiosity. Because they constantly need to be entertained. And it's affecting development at its core.

SG: It's definitely not easy to parent these days, or constantly control our growing kids' use of technology. Most parents are overstretched and some have very little support. The tablet becomes the "safe sitter," in a way. Knowing this, how can young people find a sense of purpose and sense of self when they haven't pushed their physical and psychological limits?

MS: The short answer is they can't. Purpose and sense of self come with real-world interaction. That's how you learn the boundaries of physics, the boundaries of nature. You also need to learn emotional boundaries, with and without the guidance of parents. If parents are too omnipresent, children don't learn the subtle boundaries of what hurts for others. But they're very aware of what hurts them. I think you need to give children a slightly wider berth to explore boundaries of emotionality, to make a few mistakes so they learn to correct them without parental, guardian, or teacher interference.

Now, I'm not saying, for example, that we should let bullying run rampant, but we need children to read facial expressions and signals—which is greatly compromised on and through screens—and we need them to learn empathy amongst themselves. After which parents can come in with some extra coaching when they essentially fail their own little interpersonal lessons. This natural process does not happen with screen-based technologies.

SG: Can technology interfere in the process of self-discovery?

MS: I think it thwarts it completely. Very little that you do online has anything to do with self-discovery. Even all those self-interest tests, most just want information so they can target you in advertising or maybe pick up a password or two.

The other thing about things on screens is the interaction pace. If I'm reading a book, for example, I can pause. I can put the book down and think. I can process. And I can integrate the ideas with my experience or what I've observed or that of other individuals. But when something is just presented to you, there's no reflection point. There's no time in which we can integrate information, which then turns into what we used to call wisdom.

SG: What would you tell a parent who wants to make the most informed choice when it comes to the use of technology in their household?

MS: The first thing is whatever you do or have your child do on a screen in their early years, do it with them. If you are not available and a device is available, it's absolutely basic: your child is going to learn to attach to a device. They're also going to learn their emotional regulation from a device.

If you give your young child a screen when they're having a tantrum—when they're not feeling well emotionally—they're going to learn to rely on a screen, and not a parent, to comfort themselves and to feel better. You're essentially replacing yourself. You're replacing core forms of emotional priming or emotional development with a screen. So, when a child gets a little bit older, and they're not feeling emotionally well, they're going to go to a screen, not to you, for comfort or to feel better. Similarly, when a child is bored, they're going to go to a screen, not to you or outdoors.

If a child is on a screen all the time, they're not learning to respond to their own senses or other people in a physical environment. And then we act surprised when children have trouble making friends. We act surprised when adolescents have trouble communicating. It's a complete and total set-up.

I'm sure you've noticed that we have a massive increase in impulsivity in children. So these are the kids that don't learn respect for danger. And then there's the opposite: we have a massive increase in anxiety in children. Well, that's the same issue but from the opposite side of the coin. Everything is frightening because you don't learn what isn't frightening. You don't learn that when a ladybug lands on you, it doesn't bite you. You don't learn that, with a bee you have to be a little bit cautious of it. And you definitely don't learn that if you get close to a scorpion, it will always bite you. You don't learn what is or isn't dangerous. And that affects our fight-flight-freeze response, and our attention spans, too.

Mari's words about attention span struck a chord. As someone who loves being out in nature, and who finds solace in forests and lakes and fields and fresh air, I've often wondered what we're losing as we rush through our lives in this go-go-go world. For millennia, humans lived in close connection with nature. We couldn't just rush the cycle of things, or relationships for that matter. But technology allows us to move so quickly. Without a doubt, there are upsides—getting an instant reply from a friend to a text or an email is a nice change from having to wait weeks for a letter to arrive, or even until that evening for a phone call—but what are the repercussions, for ourselves and the young people in our lives, of moving this fast? It must affect our ability to be still, to regulate our emotions, to sleep well, to make deep connections somehow? I asked Mari to weigh in on this.

63

MS: One of the key things is that technology is moving at a pace that our biology just can't keep up with. And that's why I think children, and arguably all of us, are having so much trouble.

I'm going to talk here about the attention span. You know, the increase of ADHD, etc., is in great part because most of the things we do on a screen are at such a fast pace and come with such a fast reward that the rest of life can't keep up. We're now bored unless we're at that really, really high arousal stage. But because our biology can't keep up, then we crash. So essentially, we're on a "rev, rev, rev, crash" pattern—"rev, rev, rev, crash," as opposed to much healthier cycles where the brain and the body become aroused together and then they come down together, and then they get aroused together and then they come down together.

When children are essentially functioning just at the threshold of arousal or the maximum arousal, something has to give. I call it "vestibular lock-in syndrome." That's just my name for it, but I'm sure everybody has had this experience. A child is in front of a screen. And you call them—no response. This happens because in order to pay attention to that screen, the child's threshold is at the maximum attention and—they're locked in. And what happens when that "attention lock" breaks? You have complete and total emotional deregulation. That's why they tantrum. They actually need to reboot a system that was locked that high.

That's why kids bounce off the walls when they're off their gaming devices, and the only thing that will artificially calm them again is the gaming device. But what you really need to do is kick them outside and make them run circles in the yard.

SG: Technology can be a great disruptor of natural cycles, including the circadian (sleep) cycle. Studies tell us that many of our kids are not getting enough sleep—teenagers as well. What do you have to say about this?

MS: The literature here is absolutely clear in terms of how being on our devices before bed affects melatonin production. Unfortunately, screen time is replacing snuggly time. So we're not just talking about circadian rhythm and sufficient sleep; we're talking about emotional regulation; we're talking about safety; we're talking about belonging.

Technology in the bedroom also erases intimacy. And I'm not just talking about sexual intimacy. It takes away the pillow talk. And sometimes the most important conversations between parents and children or couples is pillow talk. It's when you're quiet, when silence is not problematic—it's actually a blessing. You're in close physical proximity. You can feel breathing rate and heart rate. You're very, very in tune with each other. And, generally speaking, it is a time of extremely positive emotionality and truth talking.

SG: Best moments of my life [laughs]. Would you be willing to say that the extreme use of technology makes community more brittle?

MS: To say the least. I wouldn't even say it makes it brittle; it makes it non-existent.

SG: What happens to the brain when humans feel that there's no community?

MS: Well, we're a social species, so we feel incredibly isolated. I think that's a major contribution to our increasing complete and total lack of wellness. I think it's also probably one of the primary components in the development of depression. And if you let depression go on too long, it can also affect the body. The other thing is, we don't know how to listen anymore. We hear, but we don't know how to listen.

SG: We all need to work on this, don't we?

These are sobering words and thoughts, to be sure, but it's not all doom and gloom when it comes to tech and teens (or adults). If we talk to the young people in our lives, it becomes clear that they know

65

tech is a tool that comes with pros and cons. I asked my fifteen-year-old son, Xavier, and my fourteen-year-old daughter, Ella-Grace, about the role of social media in their lives.

Xavier told me, "Given my age, social media is a huge part of my life. While there are a lot of bad things happening on social media, it still has many benefits for our society. It's a good way to find out what's happening in the world, promote business, or plan things with friends or family. I'm a good person, but I'm not invincible, and I know that too much time spent on social media can ruin your life and show you things you don't want to see, but I think if you use it in a careful way, it can be a good thing." And Ella-Grace had this to say: "Social media is a fantastic platform for creative expression, but it can also be harmful. For instance, the effect social media has on young adults can be negative and overwhelming. Whatever your gender, sexual orientation, pronouns, or fashion choices, you will face judgment. You'll put yourself online with all the best intentions, only to be insulted and criticized arbitrarily by people you've never met. At my age, I feel as though we pay too much attention to what others think of us. This affects me, too. You only have one life, and no one out there on social media should make you feel bad about yourself, because at the end of the day, who cares!"

Yeah! I guess I've done something right? Except I still have to remind them—hundreds of times, it seems—to not be glued to their phones and to never bring them to the kitchen table. I also see them struggle with their own sense of self as they compare themselves with strangers (mostly celebrities) whom they have been taught to admire and who don't model behaviours of self-compassion and self-acceptance.

Although there is a copious amount of negativity around the use of social media and how it can affect our brains and behaviours, there is also reassuring news from the tech sector itself, where people are doing the good work of trying to make technology friendlier and safer to use. The Center for Humane Technology, for example, pictures a world in which technology "respects our attention, improves our well-being, and strengthens community." Former Google design ethicist Tristan Harris and his team have sparked the Time Well Spent movement. Harris knows that "technology is the most invisible and important political actor in the world . . . It's playing chess with your mind and it's winning every time." The centre's website includes some excellent resources to help better understand the ups and downs of tech use, to establish limits, and to explore how we can use social media and other forms of technology to build bridges instead of walls.

When I think back on my own teen years—with all of their ups and downs—I can appreciate not only the struggles that I went through but also how difficult it must have been, at times, for my parents. Raising children is hard. Raising teens can be even harder. But it's worth remembering that parents are not alone on this journey. Teens are community members, just like the rest of us, and it's in everyone's interest to make sure that they feel they have a voice, and spaces where it is safe to learn and grow. Do you cross paths with teens in your life? Perhaps you're a teacher or a coach, or maybe you work or volunteer in a place where young people hang out. If so, keep an eye open for ways to interact with these growing and changing humans. They'll benefit from your attention—and you may find that you benefit from theirs.

"Dear Diary":
Writing about Your Emotions

Whether you're a teen or the parent of a teen, or have cherished teens in your life, it's easy to sometimes feel overwhelmed by the big emotions that are such a hallmark of these turbulent years. Feeling them is difficult, but so is being on the receiving end when someone lashes out, either in person or on social media. I've learned that when you're feeling overwhelmed, there is a more effective way of dealing with it than yelling, sending an angry or criticizing text, trashing someone on social media, or just feeling like trash yourself. And it even has the benefit of being low-tech, which encourages us to step away from our devices (seriously, put that phone or tablet somewhere you can't see it). You can try this yourself, or encourage your teen to give it a shot.

First, get up from your couch or bed or desk and treat yourself to five minutes of fresh air. Then grab a pen and your journal—or any piece of paper—and start writing. Don't worry about being neat or crafting beautiful sentences. Just do it. The act of putting your feelings down on paper can seem insignificant, but it's really not. The effects of writing as a tool for healing are well-documented. Expressive writing can reduce stress, anxiety, and depression. It can improve our sleep and performance and bring us greater focus and clarity. It can help to improve immune function, since it has been shown to improve liver and lung function and help promote healing. And it can strengthen emotional functions, since it unlocks and engages right-brain creativity and gives you access to your full-on brainpower. With all of that going for it, it's worth a try!

There isn't a right or wrong way to journal about your moods or emotions. In fact, if you type "keeping a mood journal" into a search engine, you'll find tons of advice on how to get started. One option is to take a "Dear Diary" approach and just "freestyle"—write about your day and whatever you might need to get off your chest. A more focused approach is to start with whatever emotion you are feeling and then work through the situation that caused it and your response. The following prompts can get you started with this technique:

EMOTION: Name the emotion or mood you want to write about (for example, joy, fear, shame, anger, surprise, sadness, disgust).

CAUSE: Describe the event or situation that made you feel this way.

RESPONSE: Describe your response to feeling this emotion. What actions, if any, did you take?

CHECK-IN: Was the emotion an appropriate response to the situation? Did you overreact or underreact?

FOLLOW-UP: If the emotion you started with wasn't positive, what are your next steps? Is there something you can do to manage this situation, or is it a situation you need to learn to live with? If so, what coping mechanisms might help you to do that?

Try a few different approaches until you find one that works for you. And don't be surprised if you end up really looking forward to the quiet, reflective time you spend with your journal.

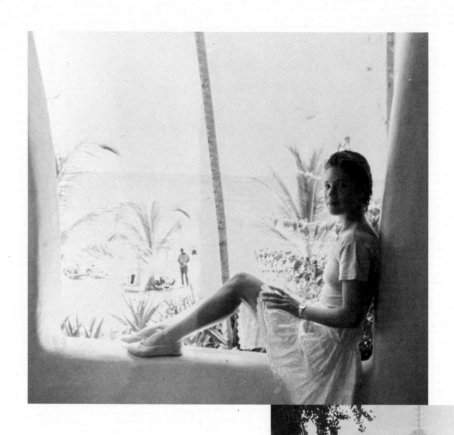

3

Culture Shock

Coming of Age in a Chaotic World

I've always done whatever I want and always been exactly who I am.

BILLIE EILISH

I t is May 22, 2022. I'm sitting at the dining room table with my cousin, her two young kids, and my whole family. Ella has two of her best friends at the table as well. Between thirteen and fourteen years old, the three of them have spent the weekend at our place. We're at the cottage and have been doing all sorts of water sports, and arts and crafts, and they had a dance party in the kitchen and built a fort.

They are adorable souls. I love meeting my kids' friends, and I feel lucky to have honest discussions with them, with lots of laughter and self-deprecation. At one point during lunch on that rainy Sunday, I tell

Ella's friends that I'm writing a book. They ask me what it's about, and I tell them: my mental health journey and how it brought me to where I am, and with experts weighing in to help the reader determine their own emotional signature and patterns. Both of them tell me: "OMG, really, I'll read it!" I immediately start weeping (which comes as no surprise to my own family members). It feels like we have already established a connection of trust, and that means so much to me.

A couple of hours later, while we are playing a game of Scrabble, I ask one of Ella's friends if she enjoys being an only child. I immediately see some sadness in her eyes and reach out my hand to hers. She is a bright, loved, creative, and talented young woman, but that doesn't mean she is without struggles. We speak of the pressures of being an only child—the pressure to perform, to please our parents, to pretend that we don't feel lonely growing up without the presence of another young person in our home. Of course, this loneliness can also be felt in a family with multiple children, and sibling rivalry is its own form of pressure. But in that moment, the child in me feels the pain in her, and that connection in itself is a gift. We all have traumas, some of the little-t variety and some bigger, and there is strength in sharing.

Like all teenagers, these girls each face their own struggles as they cope with all of the challenges that can come at this time of life and in this chaotic world of ours. Teens today are sorting out plans for their education and work life, figuring out their sexual orientation and getting to know who they are at their core, navigating the minefield that is social media, and coping with well-being and mental health challenges such as bullying, obsession with physical appearance, eating disorders, depression, cutting, and suicidal ideation—that's a lot on their plates, and in their minds. When I asked Ella-Grace if she was bothered, scared, or disturbed by anything she heard or saw at school, in movies, or on social media, she responded, "Nothing really shocks me, Mom."

While I was happy to hear that my feisty, bright, and sensitive teen is taking the messiness of her world in stride, I also couldn't (still can't) shake the familiar parental worry that comes with trying to help our children steer their way safely down what can certainly be a bumpy road. My own teen years were filled with so many wonderful moments—friends and family, school and athletic achievements, first crushes and first loves—but I also struggled to figure out who I was and how I fit into the world around me, a world that was telling me how to look and how to be in order to be beautiful and popular and happy. And that was before anyone had even heard of "social media" or "selfies."

There's no question that teenagers can feel overwhelmed by their own state of being and feeling. And when you're parenting a teenager, you, too, have to face new emotional realities and learn to better understand your child in this exciting but challenging part of their lives (and yours). Buckle up!

Testing the Waters

Have you seen the movie *Elvis*? Austin Butler does an absolutely amazing job of conveying the King's magnetic and suggestive on-stage presence, and director Baz Luhrmann accurately captures the over-the-top audience response that was such a notable feature of Elvis's performances. The way young women watched him perform was something to see: their reactions to his thrusting hips and seductive eyes, and to the music itself, was ecstatic in the true sense of the word. Back then, the dominant culture didn't celebrate women's sexual and sensuous energy, nor did people talk about desires and the need to change a system that kept women at home raising kids while it sent men out to explore their career paths. Those girls who watched Elvis on stage got a taste of sensations and emotions that were, for many, entirely unfamiliar. In this way, his music and performances opened a door to liberation. I can only imagine what that must have felt like for some of those young women. The ability to own and express our feelings and desires, and to build intimacy with ourselves and others, is a true gift.

As with so much else in life, the foundations for our relationship with our own body—and all that entails in terms of sexuality, sensuality, and body image—is formed during our early years. Think back to your own teen years for a moment. Who talked to you about how your body would transform? Who sat with you and explored the new feelings and emotions you were going to experience, or the new temptations that would cross your path as the boundaries of your world stretched beyond your home and school? How were sexuality and nudity discussed and experienced in your home?

Chances are you experienced a whole melting pot of emotions related to sensuality and sexuality during that time in your life. You may not have had the maturity to name them all, but you likely felt love, lust, infatuation, passion, and more. Too many of us are raised to be ashamed of these feelings and to suppress them. When this happens, a dangerous cycle of repression begins, and it has the potential to feed a sense of shame or even trauma that can last a lifetime if not addressed properly.

As psychotherapist and author Esther Perel wrote, there is an erotic intelligence in all of us. Her work shares profound wisdom when it comes to our desires, our cultural beliefs, and the ways in which we express ourselves sexually in our relationships. There is still so much to learn about ourselves in this area. Just like logic, rational thinking, and deep thought, erotic intelligence is another way of expressing a type of knowing, creativity, and psychological flexibility. As with the body, if the mind becomes too stiff, it will break or become fixed, and if it's overly flexible and all over the place, a sense of disorientation can set in. Talking to the young people in our lives about what they are thinking and feeling when it comes to their bodies and feelings is an important first step on the road to building erotic intelligence. And it's really never too early to begin—because we are sensual beings right from the start.

From a very young age, two things were absolutely clear to me. One was that I had both masculine and feminine energy dancing inside of me (although I couldn't have expressed it that way at the time), and the other was that I was mostly physically attracted to boys. My mom still jokes that I had my head turned toward all the blue blankets in the nursery at the hospital! As I grew up, though, it became

74

clearer to me that my fascination with boys was more than just a simple attraction. I remember being in awe of them—their easy grace and athleticism, their fearless embrace of challenges and risks, their loud enthusiasm, their confidence. I had some of that energy coursing through my own body and wanted to be able to express it as readily as they did. And, sure, okay, they weren't hard to look at, either.

Like so many of my friends, I was eager to experience a romantic relationship, with all that entailed. I would practise kissing in bed at night, pretending my hand was the face of my latest crush. I had seen some erotic pictures from pornographic magazines being swept by the wind down my street one day. Those images aroused something in me, but their rawness also made me feel uneasy. There was something so inauthentic about them, something I couldn't explain properly then.

Our sensual and sexual feelings are what they are and should never be repressed. We are all created by sex, and nothing about a healthy sexual appetite or explorations should make us feel guilty or shameful. There are so many new ways to describe what we want and what makes us happy. This is wonderful. It's helping our young people to accept their desires and fantasies, and to understand that there's no such thing as one-size-fits-all when it comes to sexuality or sensuality.

Unfortunately—and contrary to the way in which Justin and I raise our kids—these issues were never discussed in my childhood home. Yes, there were the inevitable chats about periods and contraception use, held exclusively with my mother, but that was about it. My mom could be talkative when questioned, but I sensed she was more worried for me than anything else. I also picked up on an unhealthy tension between my parents on that level. To me, sensuality and sexuality were a form of artful expression. I admired those who exuded an openness and appreciation for the beauty of bodies meeting. And yet no one in my immediate family seemed to feel the same way, or to be open to discussing these things.

One fall weekend, when I was in my early teens, my mom asked if I wanted her to purchase a book about sex and the body. She had found some magazine clippings of women in their underwear and bras that I'd hidden in my drawer. I felt a bit stupid and ashamed and told her I didn't need a book. I was quite at ease discussing sexual matters with friends, straight and gay, and nothing felt taboo to me. I was curious and quite open-minded. I wanted to learn, to explore, to test my boundaries.

I did this in the typical ways for someone my age at the time. I enjoyed swimming, and my parents made it mandatory that I take lessons at the community pool during the summer. I remember freezing every morning when my group went into the water, but I was a natural swimmer, so I stayed with it all the way through the Bronze Medallion course. There, I met a very nice, bright, and funny guy named Allen. We bonded easily and he made the lessons more fun. My other incentive to attend class was a teacher named Mark, who was a medical student. He was cute and deeply smart. I was obviously *way* too young for him, but I didn't think he was too old for me. I don't quite know what kind of victory lap I had the illusion of swimming, but I fantasized about it a thousand times over in different contexts.

I also found fodder for my imagination during weekend ski lessons at Mont-Gabriel in the Laurentians. I was part of the Thunderbirds program and rode to the mountain with other students in a big yellow school bus. Back on the bus after a long day on the slopes, with the windows fogged up from our damp clothes, I would lay my head to the side and try to gaze out the window. I sometimes pretended to fall asleep so that the counsellor I found so attractive would notice my elongated neck. I laugh so hard thinking about it now!

In case you think I was always walking around daydreaming about romantic relationships with the boys in my life, I should add that I had the privilege of experiencing many wonderful platonic friendships. I learned that if I kept conversations sincere and directly addressed any sensual or sexual tension, then it was possible to move to a level where a strong bond of trust was formed. There is nothing shameful about that tension per se; it's how you deal with it, de-dramatize it, and discuss it that allows you to tame it, if needed.

The same is true with most feelings and emotions—if we address them honestly and directly, we are always better off. To this day, I've kept wonderful and enriching long-term friendships with men in my life, and I value them deeply.

The Struggle for Control

It's amazing to me how many early memories I can call up that are related to body image. Those thoughts and feelings actually start long before our teen years. If you look at old childhood pictures of me, you'll notice that I had a bit of a boyish look. My mom kept my hair short and, thanks to my curls, it took forever to grow. I was mistaken for a boy by strangers on occasion, which didn't sit very well with me at that time. In primary school, I'd had a short bob of frizzy golden hair with bangs, and my entire face would flush anytime boys made comments on my appearance. I was one of the few girls to develop breasts early, and when playing dodge ball, some boys would throw the rubber ball hard at our chests, just to get a reaction.

It's hard to know just when I decided I needed to "do something" about my body, instead of just celebrating it for the wonderful, versatile machine that it was. I have clear images of my dad teaching me how to jump (sometimes naked) into cold lakes in every season—no shame at all. Nudity wasn't a big issue in my home. I felt a sense of pride in being athletic, and although my dad never said anything directly about my appearance, my mom would relate his occasional comments about how beautifully fit I was, and it made me feel like a million bucks. But I know now that those compliments—and so many others from so many people who felt they had a right to assess and then talk about how I looked—contributed to the pressure I put on myself to maintain my proportions. My very pretty mother was quite petite and had a tiny frame, and it was clear to me that fat on a woman was seen as unattractive. I learned very early that while boys and men were expected to "buff up," girls and women had to be thin

77

to be beautiful (but the bigger the breasts, the better). This was, after all, an era when supermodels and even porn stars, with their far-from-average bodies, were revered.

So little has changed. As I write this, "super-skinny" is making a partial comeback on the catwalk, and there's a trickle-down effect. Most bodies we see in social media, mainstream culture, and pornography are increasingly unrealistic, thanks to cosmetic surgeries that can alter us from head to toe, including our genitals. Although fashion has succeeded in putting more diverse bodies on the runway and in ads, the hot trends, as I write this in 2023, are clothes that reveal everything from the underboob to the pelvic bone, and the oversized or "off body" look where giant clothes are worn on tiny bodies. A much-hyped diabetes drug has been repurposed for weight loss under a different brand name, and the latest "must have" in plastic surgery is buccal fat removal (where fat is removed from our cheeks) to create more "chiselled" features. Where are we headed with all of this? One thing's for sure: it's not making us feel any more at ease in our natural bodies, which are beautiful just the way they are. The game of comparison and defying aging can be very dangerous and pervasive.

I grew up with the same pressure to keep thin and fit that so many young people today feel. Like any normal growing kid or teenager, I always seemed to be hungry. Our pantry at home was stocked with healthy food, and the most sugary treats I could find were ginger ale and Dad's oatmeal cookies. (The brand wore its name right: they were my dad's favourite snack, and I learned some twenty-five years later that they were also a special treat for my late father-in-law, Pierre Elliott Trudeau.) Breakfast and dinner were usually light portions, and I often felt hungry again an hour after a meal. I seemed to have the urge to eat more when I was by myself in the house. Soon, I was letting myself consume as much as I wanted. The freedom I felt when I allowed myself to eat butter-honey toast, cereal, cookies, and more might have been, in part, a response to the control my mother imposed on herself when it came to food (and then passed on indirectly to me). I wanted to eat, but I also didn't want to gain weight. My stomach would fill up quickly, and I'd be left with a feeling of slight nausea. I learned that the quickest way to get rid of that feeling was by purging. Although sticking my fingers down the back of my throat wasn't a comfortable gesture, and was one I was ashamed of, the release I would get from emptying my oversatiated stomach was greater than the cost. It was almost as if I were releasing the tight hold I felt the adults in my life had on me, and the pressures that kept building. It somehow satisfied my thirst for freedom—my thirst to be the real me, without feeling I had to fit in at every step.

By the time I hit high school, I was, like many teenagers, obsessed with physical appearance. Unfortunately, I got lots of positive re-inforcement when I kept my weight on the low side, so I internalized that concept and the pressure that accompanied it. I hid from the outside world, and bathrooms became a twisted safe haven.

I can still remember the day my parents told me they were taking me on my first (and last) trip to Europe in their company, which would include a stay in Paris, the City of Lights. I was so excited. I only wish I'd been able to leave my eating disorder at home.

I have some wonderful memories of that trip, including dancing with my father on a balcony at sunset, and meeting a lovely elderly gentleman who became a cherished pen pal. But I can also recall moments that make me feel sad for myself and wish that I'd been able to speak out about just how much I was suffering. We ate a lot of seafood during our stay, but one meal was meat-focused. That night, I didn't hold back; I ate everything I wanted. It tasted so good and I couldn't stop myself. I ate so much that I almost immediately felt overly full. Soon enough, I headed for the restrooms. There was only an open curtain partially covering the stall doors, and because those were in clear view from our table, and because the stall doors didn't make it all the way to the floor, it meant that you could see the occupant's feet. I remember thinking my parents might notice, if they looked carefully, that mine were facing the toilet bowl instead of the door. To avoid having to explain this, and feeling a lot of guilt and shame, I left my feet facing the door and twisted my entire upper body over the bowl so I could purge. I remember feeling like I was watching myself perform this contortion from a distance, but I had no control over it.

That feeling wasn't entirely new. I recall more than once observing myself in this way, as if what was happening wasn't really happening to me. But it was. My parents and I shared a scale placed in a tiny closet near my bedroom. I would weigh myself every morning and every night. I even stepped on it before and after meals. I wanted to see how I could, on my own, affect my body (my life) and be in control. At five foot five, I hit 105 pounds at my lowest, which was not healthy. I started noticing light lanugo on the sides of my face (the soft, feathery hair that helps newborns stay warm), and my periods became infrequent. This wasn't just a bit of purging when I'd overeaten. There was no question that I was suffering from a full-blown eating disorder.

Research tells us that anorexia, bulimia, and other eating disorders are not a choice; they are mental illnesses that don't discriminate (see the Selected Notes section for this chapter, page 290, for some recent studies). They affect all genders, ages, identities (racial, ethnic, sexual), and socio-economic backgrounds. They affect every organ system in the body and also have the highest death rate of any mental illness, with one in ten dying as a result of their disorder. They are caused by a combination of factors such as low self-esteem, anxiety, loneliness, personal relationship to body and food, and external environmental factors such as family dynamics and social groups. Without knowing it, I was ticking off all of those boxes. I was a strong-willed, courageous, and sensitive young woman, and yet I felt lost at times. The truth is that many mental illnesses are a defence response to uncertainty. Food became my "drug of reassurance," the way I told myself that everything would be okay. I couldn't save my parents from their pain, I couldn't control whatever was going on between them, I couldn't help my father through his addiction and emotional withdrawal, so I had to find certainty somewhere. It was obviously false certainty, but one uses the tools at one's disposal.

By the time I was in my late teens, I was adept at hiding my eating disorder. My parents and closest friends had no idea. My boyfriend was only just beginning to get suspicious. Only my best friend knew. She listened to me without judgment but couldn't understand why I was doing it. She was struggling with her own body issues in other ways, so neither of us was equipped to truly help the other. Then, one night during my second year in CEGEP (Quebec junior college), everything changed. I was lying in bed, crying and trembling. I was feeling lost, sad, out of control, angry, confused, and scared. I'd purged too much and for too long that evening, and it had left me shaken. That's when I heard my mom preparing for bed in the bathroom right beside my room. A voice somewhere deep inside was urging me to ask for help, to share my angst, to relieve myself from all the unwanted stress I was bottling up (and purging). In that instant, I softly cried out, "*Maman?*"

It took her all of six seconds to arrive by my bedside. She knew by the tone of my voice that something was off. She sat on my bed and I asked her to lie down. She asked me what was going on, and for once, I didn't hold back. I told her that something was wrong, that I wasn't doing well and couldn't go on like this. I took a deep breath and finally said the words out loud: "I have an eating disorder and I need help. I need your help."

She was immediately reassuring and admitted that she'd suspected something but had never been sure. She said she was sorry. I felt relieved but also angry and sad. Why hadn't she tried to reach out to me sooner? I knew very well that she'd noticed I was losing weight, because she had commented on it. The problem was that some of her comments had been almost reinforcing. My mom, like so many women of that time (and still), had completely bought into the idealized notions of feminine beauty. In that moment, though, those thoughts took a back seat to worry. How would my mom present all this suffering of mine to my dad? What would he think? And how was all of this going to work out, now that I'd told someone?

My mom told my father that I was suffering from an eating disorder and that I needed help. He took the news calmly and with sadness. At the time, he sat on the board of the Sainte-Justine hospital and the

Cachou Tournament, which raised funds for sick kids, and he didn't waste any time asking his friends about which doctors were best to see for eating disorders. On my first visit to the doctor, I was interviewed by an intern who asked questions about my life and how I felt about myself. I remember them commenting on the fact that my thighs weren't fat at all. Bizarrely, it made me feel better. I guess I also had body dysmorphia issues and, like many other patients, wasn't seeing my body as it actually was. I also began therapy with a psychologist, which seemed to help.

My father never spoke directly to me about my eating disorder—not then or at any other time during my life. I always wondered why. It made me sad, and I felt abandoned in a way, because I interpreted his distance as indifference. I now understand that it was too much for him to handle. He knew nothing about eating disorders and was already dealing with his own struggles, which he never spoke of to me. I wish he had. To this day, I'm still trying to understand him better. He's my dad, and I love him.

When I look back at some of my most challenging teenage and young adult days, it's almost as if I can see my adult self standing right beside me. Oh, if only she'd been able to share some of her hard-earned wisdom! So many of us were starving ourselves to be thin, and therefore to be admired and loved. I feel almost sick as I write that now, and the behaviour was certainly making us sick then. I wish we'd been able to talk openly about what we were experiencing and the impossible supermodel standards we were trying to live up to. Instead, we admired and judged each other from afar, focusing mostly on exterior attributes.

In high school, there were a couple of older girls I looked up to. Most of them had a natural beauty and were athletic. There was one girl in particular whom I recall: she drove a Jeep, and I thought she was so cool. We never really got to know each other, though. Imagine my surprise, then, when I was watching TV one day, more than twenty years later, and saw her on a show where eating disorders were being discussed. She'd become a psychologist and was, like me, trying to get honest conversations about eating disorders started with the public. We've since reconnected and collaborated on a few different occasions.

Dr. Stéphanie Léonard specializes in the treatment of eating disorders, eating behaviours, and body image. She is the author of *Mirror Mirror: Living with Your Body*, and the founder of Bien Avec Mon Corps, an organization whose mission is to promote a healthy body image and positive self-esteem in young people. She told me that millions of North Americans were suffering from eating disorders before the pandemic, and that the numbers have risen steeply since. Part of this may be due to the increased use of social media during these challenging times. Studies have shown us that the use of social media is associated with greater body dissatisfaction, a distorted body image, a negative perception of our own physical attributes, a tendency to compare ourselves to others, the internalization of unrealistic beauty norms, and—you guessed it—an increased risk of developing an eating disorder in vulnerable people. I started my conversation with Stéphanie by asking her why she decided to focus on eating disorders in her practice.

Dr. Stéphanie Léonard: Like you, and with you, I went to an all-girls school, and I was astonished by the number of girls who were suffering from them. Some of them were fainting in gym class or had all sorts of very specific behaviours around food. Others were engaging in self-induced vomiting. I wanted to understand why this illness was hitting some girls and not others.

Sophie Grégoire: Sometimes it feels like we've been taught to be at war with our own bodies. We hate our bodies to the point of changing their shape, proportions, and size. How do we swim against this strong current?

SL: It starts with all the little things we do in a day—to assert ourselves with the people we love, to be able to express our needs, to be able to open up when we are suffering, to be able to make mistakes and be kind to ourselves anyway.

I also think it starts with authenticity and self-knowledge, and maybe being lucky enough to grow up in an environment where the adults around you provide an effective mirror, so you are able to explore, see, and recognize your strengths and your challenges, engage in trial and error, and feel you can be authentic and discover who you truly are. Providing a mirror means that children feel safe to be themselves, knowing there is an unconditional presence or support behind them.

As adults, we need to meet our children where they are, because they can be very different from us, and we shouldn't make assumptions; we need to ask questions. Unfortunately, at this moment, social media is partly raising our children. They spend much more time with it than with us, with their family, or even sometimes with their friends, even though they communicate. So it has become a mixed space for me. There are super-inspiring things, and then there are highly toxic and unregulated things, making it chaotic. Young people learn to live waiting for feedback from other people and the world. It's harmful.

SG: In adolescence, young people's bodies are in turmoil and intense transformation. It's not easy to deal with all of these changes.

SL: It's complicated because teens don't all react the same way. We know that at age five, children start to be concerned about their physical appearance. It depends on who you are, your temperament, your background, and the changes you are going through. Having pimples, gaining weight, witnessing your body changing, that's normal, but there is also a big gap between the changes that occur and what teens see as models for beauty they are supposed to resemble. For boys, it's different, because there is pressure for them to be big, to have an athletic body, to be slim, to be symmetrical in their features. In Quebec, half of teens don't like their physical appearance, boys and girls combined. Before, there were always two sets of statistics, one for girls, one for boys. Now, it seems the boys have caught up to the girls.

SG: As you know, I suffered from eating disorders. With time, I realized that food wasn't the problem. It became my drug of choice—like alcohol or gaming or sex, etc. So what can cause an eating disorder?

SL: For a long time, we thought it was difficult family environments, perfectionist personality traits, rigidity, and all that. While these factors can play a role, we now know that there is a significant genetic basis for the risk of developing an eating disorder. In other words, it's a vulnerability. To develop an eating disorder, there has to be a genetic vulnerability that is triggered, or not, through your life experiences and environment. Our culture's obsession with youth and the body doesn't help either.

SG: What are the major warning signs?

SL: There are medical conditions that come with food restriction or self-induced vomiting, taking laxatives, fasting, or using enemas. There are signs to watch for: Menstruation may diminish or stop completely. There may be hair loss or dry skin. The body can be covered in a fine hair called lanugo. Tooth enamel can be affected, and gastrointestinal problems can occur. Your body, physically, is speaking to you, but emotionally, when it gets to the point that it takes so much space that it is a constant source of anxiety and inner debate, it's like having a huge ink stain on your life. There can be a desire for perfection, withdrawal from social life, extreme diets, a lack of interest in activities that used to be enjoyable, even a sense of despair. People confide in others less and withdraw. Behaviour before and after a meal has to be considered—if the person goes to the bathroom frequently during or after the meal.

We have to look closely and listen, without judgment. We need to remember that the person feels isolated with this illness. It's like finding yourself behind a glass wall with your life unfolding on the other side, in front of your eyes, but you don't really have access to it. When you are in the grips of an eating disorder or any sort of compulsion, you think you are feeling everything, but you are preventing yourself from feeling, and when you stop yourself from feeling, anxiety mounts, and you detach from what you are, and then you can stumble and sink into depression.

SG: Through culture and social media, we often get messages such as "You're not beautiful the way you are. Only young people are beautiful." Or we get told, "Oh, you don't age; you're so beautiful." Can those dehumanizing messages make us sick?

SL: In fact, that's what uproots us completely from our uniqueness and who we are fundamentally. We are obsessed with this image that is outside us and that we think we have to fit. There is insidious conditioning going on in the way we perceive and feel, and it starts early, with toys children play with and the comments they hear. We are trained to like certain features, trained to like looking at what is skinny, to like smooth, unwrinkled skin.

Some people manage better than others, but I think it's the source of a great deal of human suffering among young people and adults, too. It can instill a real feeling of panic. We must realize what is intuitive, what is natural, what is in our genes without having it be short-circuited or modified. It's like our pure essence cannot exist in peace. I remember a young girl in a school I visited who told me, "Madame, surgery bothers me, because I don't know what a woman who is forty, fifty, or sixty is supposed to look like anymore!"

We have lost respect for aging, recognizing the positive sides of aging, the wisdom we gain. It is a natural process that is so enriching for the individual and society, but it is completely demonized, and we are afraid and sow doubt within ourselves. That doubt then gets manifested physically in changes we make to our faces and bodies. And worse yet, we convince ourselves that we are doing it for ourselves and to build our self-esteem.

SG: Do you think our culture encourages the space needed to explore oneself and connect with new experiences?

SL: That's a very good question. Our individualistic, performance-oriented world makes so many people unhappy, because we want young people to fit a mould. Fortunately, we are starting to deconstruct false beliefs that can make it such that young people don't feel okay, whether in terms of sexual orientation or in terms of body diversity—all sorts of things. But there is more work to be done. We are in reaction mode when teens do things that we think are unsuitable, but were we listening beforehand, and are we giving them space? I think there are settings where for some people, it's just too much, and they can't slow down to ask questions, because they are in emotional survival mode.

SG: Wouldn't it be better for all of us to really sit with whatever is causing us to suffer and look deeper within ourselves, rather than detaching from that suffering?

SL: Exactly. I always say there are several areas to work on with an eating disorder: there's nutritional rehabilitation, body image, and then there's how the disorder has become an adaptative mechanism for managing emotions and self-regulation. But then we hear "Well, it helps me to disconnect; it helps me not feel." While you are doing that, though, it doesn't go away, and as soon as you open that door, you feel like it's a tsunami hitting you, because you are facing an accumulation of suffering. It's uncomfortable to confront yourself when for years you have sort of surfed on top of your emotions.

But at a certain point, you learn to tame them, and you experience small victories. It's tempting to try to work only on the "unhealthy" voice of the illness, but you also have to strengthen the healthy voice. That's the one that at certain points will say, "Okay, I really don't feel good. I will tolerate. I will wait a bit. I will let the wave go by . . . It will pass." In this way, you patiently regain control of your emotions.

Eating Disorders: Know What to Look for, Know What to Ask

You may not think you know anyone who has struggled with an eating disorder, but chances are you do. According to the National Initiative for Eating Disorders, more than one in five Canadian teenagers are on a diet at any given time, which puts them at risk for an eating disorder. Many people with an eating disorder don't get diagnosed, which means the real numbers are hard to know.

There are three major families of eating disorders—anorexia nervosa, bulimia nervosa, and binge eating disorder—as well as orthorexia and bigorexia. Here's a quick breakdown:

ANOREXIA NERVOSA causes an obsession with weight and food, and can create a distorted body image (for example, you may see yourself as "fat," even though your weight is very low). To cope with the stress, anxiety, and low self-esteem that come as a result of this distorted body image, sufferers may restrict food intake and become fixated on burning calories through physical activity. These activities may offer a sense of control.

BULIMIA NERVOSA is characterized by binge eating (eating a large amount of food in a short period of time) and episodes of purging (vomiting or using laxatives) or fasting.

BINGE EATING DISORDER is similar to bulimia nervosa, but without compensatory behaviours.

BIGOREXIA is a dependence on physical activity that interferes with other aspects of your life. Those who suffer from this disorder are often very strict with their diet and workout plan and may take supplements and steroids.

ORTHOREXIA is an overwhelming concern with healthy eating. It often begins with the elimination of certain foods—white flour, refined sugar, red meat, alcohol, for example—and then snowballs. Social activities often disappear, because it's too challenging to figure out what to eat at a restaurant or friend's house, and weight loss often occurs.

The good news is that with early detection and intervention, a full recovery is possible (I know this first-hand). If you are concerned about yourself or about a young person in your life, Dr. Stéphanie Léonard suggests asking a few questions to determine whether you should reach out for help:

- Do I spend lots of time trying to control what I eat and manage my weight?
- Am I critical of my physical appearance?
- Am I spending a lot of time comparing myself with others?
- Do I ever feel ashamed or disgusted by my own body?
- Do I feel guilty when I'm under the impression that I'm not enough in control of my diet and my body?

Identity Crisis

It was so interesting to speak with Stéphanie Léonard about the dangers of social media when it comes to body image. Over the past several years, I've seen that play out in my own life. I have a front-row seat to the hateful comments directed at public figures through social media channels. As a politician, Justin has been a constant recipient, as have other members of Parliament. Female cabinet ministers, in particular, have suffered online abuse. So many of these incredibly talented, intelligent, hard-working women have received indecent, misogynist, disrespectful, and degrading comments on their looks, their femininity, and their work. Sometimes the abuse even extends to death threats. It's happened to me, too. While hosting or conducting interviews live on Instagram, even as public personalities are confiding their mental health struggles, unwelcome comments appear on my screen. "If I was married to her, I'd tell her to get breast implants," one will say; another, that the father of my children "should rot in jail"—all while I'm trying to shed light on deeply important issues and incredible life stories. It's just so concerning and sad, even for the abusers.

I've learned that I can stop those comments from appearing on my screen with the push of a button, which is helpful, but I'd be lying if I said the constant insults and lies don't get to me. And I'm an adult. What does the constant judgment, the instant feedback, and the in-the-moment stimulation do to our teenagers, whose brains and ability to think critically are still developing? And what effect does all of that noise have on our sense of who we are, and the ways we imagine we "fit," or don't, into the world around us?

Earlier in this chapter, I shared some of the ways I'd internalized the messages I saw and heard about what was considered attractive, and how I knew from a very early age that there was a core part of me that possessed what would typically have been thought of as "male" energy. I also recall feeling somehow ashamed of, or punished by society for, the true strength of my gender, sexuality, and sensuality. Although I couldn't identify with many of her more "out there" behaviours, I idolized Madonna for her freedom of expression, male-female energy, and the ways in which she defied norms. I felt like I was living in a world (and sometimes a family and a community) with double standards. Most men wanted their daughters to be fierce and courageous, but their wives to be more obedient and at their service in some pernicious ways. So I felt I had to be all of those things at once.

As we discussed with Stéphanie Léonard, social media has muddied the waters on these issues and others around identity in dangerous ways. We've bestowed über-celebrity status on women who present unnatural and unattainable beauty standards to the world. Endless selfies—taken with just the right light and perfected with filters—are shared. And influencers know just how to pose to make their waists look tiny or their muscles (or breasts) look big. This has a profound negative impact on the emotional and mental well-being of our young people. Younger and younger women are using chemicals or needles on their faces and plastic surgery on various parts of their bodies, and boys are taking supplements to help them look like the built-up guys they see online. With all of this pressure to conform, it's no wonder so many of us are anxious, exhausted, afraid, and depressed.

There is, though, some cause for hope. I see Ella and her friends looking at models strutting their stuff with more discernment than I had at their age. I'm grateful for that, but we risk making a grave mistake if we focus only on young women when we talk about the pressures to conform to traditional notions of beauty and behaviour. Our boys are feeling that pressure, too, and the ways in which that plays out have huge repercussions not only for them but for our society as a whole.

Liz Plank is an award-winning Canadian journalist, host of *The Man Enough Podcast*, and bestselling author of *For the Love of Men*. Liz told me that she grew up in a family where the women experienced "trauma rooted in patriarchal violence." As I was watching a clip from her podcast, I was struck by the truth of the words and ideas she was discussing with the men around the table: "The best way a girl, woman, or daughter will learn to respect herself and learn that she's valued is if you [men/fathers] value girls, women, and their mothers." As an adult, she's become "passionate about eradicating any kind of sexism and inequality, because I saw that it was just hurting the people around me." We had a fascinating and important conversation about the connections between gender equality and mental health.

> **Sophie Grégoire:** You speak of and have researched toxic and mindful masculinity. On your podcast, you invite men to talk about this. In so many ways and for so long, men have not been given the space to live or process their true emotions—sadness, vulnerability, anger. How is that affecting the notion of masculinity and how men navigate through it all?
>
> **Liz Plank:** That's the crux of the issue of patriarchal violence in our society. And it is not just causing a lot of pain and suffering to women, which is what I saw growing up. I wasn't aware that the men that were hurting the women around me had also been hurt by the patriarchy. And that men are the first victims of the patriarchy, and then they end up often committing violence to themselves and to each other. And the flip side of that is not making space for any kind of vulnerability, any kind of feminine energy.
>
> What I have seen in the last ten years is women finally being given permission to express their masculine energy, be more assertive, be more confident, be more dominating, be more assertive, sort of put themselves out there. And what I'm hoping the next wave of feminist activism leads to is men being able to really lean into their feminine energy, which is to be more nurturing—and not just to other people, but to themselves.
>
> **SG:** We sometimes hear that men look to sex to get closer emotionally, because they don't have that emotional connection in their own friendships, because it's not something that we

support or encourage in our society. What have men told you about how these dynamics affect them?

LP: In a patriarchal society, we're more familiar with what women lose when they're objectified, when there's violence against them if they dress a certain way or express a certain kind of sexuality. And then men get punished when they're not asserting that sexual energy, and that is actually the only way that they're allowed to express emotion and connection and seek that kind of connection.

In heterosexual relationships, you have one half that's been told to be ashamed of their sexuality and only see connection through emotion. And then the other half has been told, "You can only see connection sexually, not with emotion." Put those two people together, and you have the issue that we have right now, which is not just divorce and an impact on marriage, but, in the younger generation, record levels of single people, of single men who are dissatisfied and who are saying, "I'm involuntarily celibate. I want to be with women and I can't."

But then there are also women who are voluntarily single, there's a whole femcel movement with Gen Z. Last year in the United States, more single women bought homes than single men, even though single women have a lower median income.

SG: You've had so many men from all walks of life on your podcast. Have any of them spoken about pornography and the narrow ideals that are putting so much pressure on women and on men, in different ways?

LP: We do talk a lot about porn. I think it is such a shame that porn has commodified the experience of sex, which should be the last thing that we commodify—intimacy should never be something that's commodified. There's nothing wrong with sex; it's when it becomes a whole industry and when boys and men particularly are exposed to it far too early, and to the kind of porn that's really teaching them the wrong thing, that we really get into issues.

There's a study that we talk about on the podcast, where after men have watched porn, they're more likely to see women as objects. Again, sex is great; it's the fact that in our society, we objectify women so much and there's so much violence against women that that's what happens to men's brains. When women watch porn, that doesn't happen. Women can see and have an experience, a sexual connection with a man, and not then go out in the street and think that he's lesser. I wish women could be sexual in a way that doesn't diminish their humanity [in the eyes of men].

SG: How do we as women help redefine a more mindful masculinity. What's our role?

LP: I love that question. Some women are uncomfortable with the fact that women like you and me talk about masculinity. They'll say this isn't our labour. But it's actually kind of patriarchal to be like, "You're over here; we're over there; you fix your stuff," without realizing this is my neighbour, this is my dad, this is my son. So of course we're all connected, and we need to really lean into the aspect of community—again, these sorts of feminine energy characteristics of nurturing, of community, of relatedness—and support men in the way that I think the best men support us in becoming and reaching our full potential as human beings, but as women, too.

SG: Men have told you that they are a bit anxious about asking for directions, literally and metaphorically. Who guides them, then? Or is it just a free-for-all and they're just figuring it out as they go?

LP: I think it's such a disservice that there are men out there who won't look to women as leaders in this space of challenging the status quo. Women have been really at the forefront of all revolutions, but particularly the gender revolution. I think if we didn't live in a patriarchal society, men would be looking to women in terms of modelling that kind of work. And the thing that is so unique about the way that women do it is that we do it through community. We build these circles at work and in our family lives with friendships.

SG: Are there lessons we can learn from other communities on this front?

LP: Radical acceptance is a really big one, and just doing things on your terms and reimagining . . . I was going to say reimagining the box, but there is no box. It's very freeing to queer your life.

"Queering" is a verb in feminist theory for a reason. And you can actually be queer in all these different ways, not just in the bedroom and in your romantic relationship. Queering families means it is not this nuclear box of a mom and a dad. It is a whole other way of imagining community, of imagining individuality.

Liz's thoughts on the importance of community reminded me of a conversation I had recently with Mary Simon, Canada's governor general, and the first Indigenous woman to hold that office. We'll hear more from her in chapter 8 about trauma and mental health issues in the Indigenous community, but we also spoke about the challenges of long-held notions of masculinity and the ways they can hold our boys and men back.

"Most men, they hide it," she told me, speaking about how men typically bottle up their emotions. "They've never been taught. They're told never to cry. So our concept of masculinity and manhood is flawed. To create more peace in this society, we can't push half of the population aside and keep them under their repressed emotions. There's more work to do, and we can't be like the men of the past and ignore it. We have to say to the men, 'You need to come into the fold and work with us.' We have to unite to actually plan the future."

What a lovely idea—to unite, to learn from each other, to build bridges instead of walls. Feeling like you belong to a community is viscerally reassuring and encourages a sense of safety. This makes me think of sisterhood. There's no way I would have gotten where I am today on my own path without the help of girls and women around me. On a grander scale, I've been inspired by trailblazers who have enlarged their own space of empowerment to include as many women as possible—women such as Malala Yousafzai, Amal Clooney, Hillary Rodham Clinton, Chelsea Clinton, Michelle Obama, Angela Merkel, Gloria Allred, Ruth Bader Ginsburg, Gloria Steinem, Madeleine Albright, Monica Lewinsky, and so many more who have experienced the backlash and nastiness of toxic masculinity. When I got the chance to meet or interview many of them, I realized I wasn't the only one thinking about how important it is to include men and boys in the equation for equality.

Thankfully, I have also met many inspiring men who are allies in this fight. Although too few men have role models who inspire them to work toward ending gender-based injustices, there are some good ones leading the way. The unrealistic concepts boys and young men live with when it comes to constructing their mature selves is an insult to their intelligence and true potential. Our willingness to discuss these issues with young people in our lives will help create a safe space where they can get to know themselves better. This, in turn, will help them move into adulthood with the confidence to define their own world and selves instead of giving in to distorted cultural standards.

A Patriarchy Primer

We hear a lot these days about the patriarchy and various types of masculinity, and it can be hard to stay on top of the terminology. Here, a few of the experts I've spoken to help us sort it all out:

PATRIARCHY: Oxford Languages tells us that *patriarchy* is a "system of society or government in which men hold the power and women are largely excluded from it." While the power dynamics may be working in men's favour, other things are not. Under patriarchy, men "can't feel anything vulnerable," says author Terry Real. "The more invulnerable you are the more manly you are; the more vulnerable you are the more girly you are—and that's not a good thing." He continues: "The way we 'turn boys into men' is through disconnection. We teach them to disconnect from their hearts, from their wants and needs, and from others. They are allowed two emotions: rage and lust. And all of the tender emotions are illegal."

TOXIC MASCULINITY involves the need to compete with and dominate others. "I think patriarchy is simply toxic masculinity writ large," Terry says. "Patriarchy is the code of masculinity that's now superimposed on all of us—men and women."

PRECARIOUS MASCULINITY is the idea that masculinity is something "very hard to earn but also extremely easy to lose," says Liz Plank. She compares it to an inflatable doughnut or boat: "There's a hole, and so you constantly have to blow into it and it'll stay inflated, but the minute you stop, it goes down to zero. And no matter what big masculine thing you did—if you wrestled with a bear while you were drinking a beer and eating a steak with the other hand—the next day, if you order a drink and it comes in a cosmopolitan glass, then you're not a man and you have to prove that you are."

MINDFUL MASCULINITY starts with the premise that there is no definition of masculinity. According to Liz Plank, "We've actually distorted the definition of masculinity because of patriarchy. It's giving it back to men to define and reimagine," in the same way women have been encouraged to reflect on what parts of femininity they want to embrace at different times. "It's encouraging men to have flexibility and really approach it in a mindful way."

Toxic Masculinity and Women's Health
WITH DR. GABOR MATÉ

Toxic masculinity can contribute to patriarchal and sexist behaviours that threaten women and hold them back. As Liz Plank wrote on Instagram: "Anxiety makes women suppress our needs in the service of the wants of others. The patriarchy loves a damaged woman." It's not as well known, though, that unhealthy notions of masculinity can have a negative effect on women's physical health. Dr. Gabor Maté has said that in our society, women hold the emotional load of the house. I asked him to explain that and to talk about the repercussions:

Dr. Gabor Maté: When we talk about repression of anger, and taking care of the emotional needs of others ahead of our own, and about being afraid to disappoint others . . . which gender in this culture is programmed to do that? Female. When you have a certain emotional pattern, that's going to show up in your physiology.

Women are more likely to have mental illness diagnoses and take medications for anxiety or depression than men. Also, 70 or 80 percent of autoimmune disease happens to women, like lupus, rheumatoid arthritis, multiple sclerosis, and so on. Women are also more prone to have non-smoking-related cancers. We've had multiple studies showing a relationship between stress and rheumatoid arthritis. So what are the characteristics of people with rheumatoid disease or autoimmune disease? Repression of healthy anger, being nice, helpful, taking care of others ahead of themselves. Evolution gave us these systems—immune system, nervous system, emotional system. The role of the emotional system is to allow in what is friendly and nurturing and loving, and to keep out what isn't. What's the role of the immune system?

The same. Psychoneuroimmunology studies the oneness of the immune system, the nervous system, the hormone apparatus, and the emotional system in the brain. This is all one system.

Guess what happens when you suppress your emotions? You're also messing with the immune system.

So, to go back to your question about women—women have been given this job of absorbing the stresses of everybody, and that shows up in their bodies and in their minds.

Part 2

Transitions

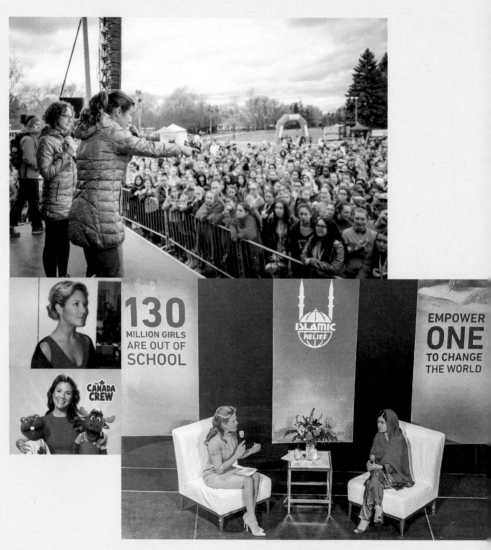

Interviewing Malala Yousafzai

4

The Winding Road

Fumbling toward Purpose

The truth will set you free, but first, it will piss you off!

GLORIA STEINEM

I can recount almost every word of the conversation my mom and I had when we were trying to figure out where I was going after CEGEP. We were sitting in the house in Sainte-Adèle, near a window, with papers piled all over the table. My mom had tried to sit me down a couple of times before as well, and the talks always went something like this: "Sophie, I'm very worried that you're going to miss some deadlines and you won't be able to get into a university of your choice. You absolutely have to fill out all these forms!" And, maybe in a slightly condescending or impatient tone, I would say something like: "Moooooom, relaaaaaaaax. It's gonna be fine. People face much more difficult problems in this world! Maybe I should take a gap year, travel and find work somewhere." But that was not a scenario my parents were willing to consider. They were protective of and concerned for their only daughter, and didn't feel it was safe to just send me out into the world all by myself. I don't remember discussing university plans with my father at all, although he was usually the one who helped me to explore by pushing my boundaries. I had hoped for his insight when it came time to fly out of the nest, but it didn't really happen—apart from him saying that studying business would be a good base from which to start.

While one stage of my life was ending, another was beginning—but I didn't have a good sense of where I was heading. I couldn't yet feel a passion that would propel me toward my future. I felt I had so much more to experience before shoving my nose in books again. And yet, that fall, I ended up doing a daily train commute with a heavy bag filled with microeconomics, statistics, and accounting books, after I'd been accepted into the commerce program at McGill University. At the end of the first semester I passed all my tests, but I definitely knew I didn't want two more years of these subjects. I switched to the Université de Montréal, where I studied industrial relations and psychology, which accumulated into a bachelor's degree in communications. I graduated with honours, but while I'd enjoyed my psychology courses and even the rigours of linguistics, that was about it. I had so much to give, but I was just buzzing around without a spot to land.

I think a lot of young people feel the same way I did. In a society that dictates how we should look, feel, and act, what does it mean to "find yourself," to discover your passion(s) and purpose? I believe it is the birthright of all human beings to be their creative selves and develop and find a sense of purpose. Unfortunately, we are not all given the same opportunities to do this, which means that many of us fumble along by trial and error. What are we to do with ourselves and our lives? Tyler Knott Gregson is an autistic photographer, writer, and poet whose work I love, and whom I had the chance to interview recently. In his newsletter, *Signal Fire*, he wrote: "[W]e all have an inner voice, it's whispering to us at all times . . . But we commit a sin when we suppress it, we hide it from ourselves, we dirty our own mirrors in order to live in that soft-haze of denial . . . It is a tragedy too of settling for less than what lights our soul on fire, of pretending that less is enough."

I agree with Tyler. We need to chase after what lights our souls on fire, and listen to what that inner voice is telling us. But slowing down enough to do that can be challenging as we emerge from those tumultuous teenage years into young adulthood. Author Brené Brown says that the opposite of belonging is fitting in. Trying to fit into any narrowing, imposing, manipulative, or coercing structures (physical or mental) betrays our authentic self. When we live in this state of hypocrisy, we don't allow ourselves to be creative. We are in resistance mode. This can affect our capacity for connection, our ability to co-operate and collaborate with friends and loved ones, the ways in which we express our unique sensuality and sexuality, our creative potential, and our sense of purpose.

In order to live a life of emotional integrity and cohesion—an authentic life—we must do the hard work of looking at the world the way it is, and also of looking at ourselves the way *we* are, with all of our qualities and flaws. These days, I find we are encouraged to know how to belong to society before we are taught how to belong to ourselves. Belonging to yourself—becoming yourself—is an act of courage and of rebellion.

A Sense of Self

Sometimes it takes just one encounter, one conversation, to give us a little nudge in the right direction. As I was still struggling to find my way during university, I held on to the memory of a bond I'd created with a total stranger a few years earlier, while still in CEGEP.

Not long after first semester began that year, I was called to the administrator's office. I had no idea why I'd been summoned, but he didn't beat around the bush. He explained that a promising new student was experiencing some difficulties integrating. As he described her struggles, I felt sad for what she had been going through. It must have shown on my face. "I can see how you're feeling, Sophie, and I think you can help her," the administrator said. I promised him I'd do my best to ease her transition. She and I talked over the phone and in person a few times about life and all its tribulations.

I think it was easy for me to relate to that young woman because I was suffering myself on a few different levels. One day not long after that meeting with the administrator, I was feeling sad, lonely, and ashamed about my ongoing struggles with food (this was still a few months before I finally got help). I went to a bathroom in a very quiet corner of the huge school building where I felt safe to relieve myself from overeating. After a meal, I would sometimes walk the hallways until I ended up in this section of the building, far from all of my classes, and I had started noticing another pair of shoes visible under one of the stall doors in my safe-spot washroom—the same shoes each time. I'd also noticed noises coming from that stall, like a paper bag crinkling.

On this particular day, I actually saw a young woman come out of the stall. In a flash, I understood what was happening. I was coming to this bathroom to get rid of my meal, but this was where she was eating hers. Not with friends in the dining hall, or even on a bench outside of a classroom, but in a bathroom stall, all alone. My heart sank. I can't remember if we exchanged pleasantries, though I think we did, but I do remember just wanting to hold her close. I made myself a few promises that day. One was that I would figure out a way, someday, to help those with struggles similar to mine. The other was that I would never overeat and purge again.

Well, I wasn't able to keep that second promise. I know now that eating disorders are a disease, a sickness, and not a character flaw. A desire to heal is important, but it isn't nearly enough. You can't just snap yourself out of a mental health issue. Like any other form of compulsion, it takes emotional awareness and literacy to get to the roots of your suffering. Nor is healing a straight line.

As for the first promise? Helping people who struggle with eating disorders and other mental health issues has become a core part of who I am. I've come to see that I am most myself when connecting with people on a deeply personal level, and I cherish the moments I get to spend doing this. Each of those connections is a gift, something that feeds my sense of purpose and brings meaning to my life. And I love how things can sometimes come full circle in the most unexpected ways. In June 2022, twenty-eight years after that day in the bathroom, I was invited back to Brébeuf to speak to some of the female students about my mental health journey. It was a very emotional homecoming, and a true honour for me to meet this remarkable group of young women (which included my beloved niece). During our visit, throughout which more than a few tears were shed, I suggested that students should have access to an "emotional library" to help them navigate the ups and downs of their lives. I asked the girls who were comfortable doing so to share the worst thing they'd ever gone through. From abuse and bullying to loss, grief, racial injustice, and acute family drama, some very sad stories were shared that day in what is considered to be a school for the privileged. It was yet another reminder that it doesn't matter where you come from; we are all just one trauma away from each other. At the end of the event, we lined up to make sure everyone got a heartfelt goodbye hug. A few days later, I received an email letting me know that the college was going to encourage the girls to build a real emotional library by having everyone share their story anonymously. This truly moved me.

I think often about those girls I met that day, and the ones I knew when I was younger who had such different personalities from me but

> *Your passion is for you and your purpose is for others. When you use your passion in the service of others, it becomes your purpose.*
>
> JAY SHETTY

with whom I shared a similar longing. We all had so much potential, but we didn't know the essential parts of ourselves yet, the parts that would help us figure out the kinds of careers, hobbies, volunteer and advocacy work, and even relationships that would be most fulfilling. What I realize now is that most young people need help and guidance on these issues, and we are not always showing up for them. Finding one's passion and transforming it into a job is a rare reality. There's no rule that says work has to define our sense of self. A healthy sense of who we are is not rooted in career choices but in personal character. Ignoring parts of ourselves in order to fit a preconceived notion of who we should be comes with risks attached. We might be wildly successful in our chosen career and still unhappy—as we try to silence a little voice inside our head or a feeling deep in our gut that's telling us something isn't right.

Katherine (Katie) Dudtschak knows all too well the cost of ignoring that little voice, as she went through a very public gender affirmation. She is a deeply experienced and respected business leader. She worked at Canada's largest bank, where she led a national team of more than twenty-five thousand advisors in branches and business centres, as well as expert advisors. Professionally and personally, she is a passionate advocate for diversity, equity, and inclusion. Under her leadership, her team made measurable gains on the inclusion and advancement of women, BIPOC, and LGBTQ+ individuals.

Making your way through your own struggles—whether it's an addiction process, a professional learning curve, a lack of purpose, or trying to figure out who you are at your core—can be a chaotic ordeal. I was struck when I heard Katie say, "I tried so hard to fit into a masculine world, because I was fearful." And yet, even in the face of that fear, she couldn't hold in who she really was. "There was a time early in my career when I skipped!" she told me. "I was in a really good mood and I skipped across the inside of the bank branch. You don't think of bankers skipping across a branch. I definitely experienced some backlash."

Living life as the truest version of yourself certainly can stir up insecurities and emotions, and it can even cause disruption around

108

you, but it's also the most enriching and liberating path. Just listen to what Katie has to say about this:

> **Sophie Grégoire:** Can you tell us more about the conflicting emotions you felt as a child, and how they came together as you grew up?
>
> **Katie Dudtschak:** I grew up in a small town, in a rural community, on a farm. I rode my bicycle over jumps, and I rode on snowmobiles and I loved snow, and I loved camping. Those things allowed me to feel like I somewhat fit in a boy's world. However, there was a pattern of feelings and behaviour as young as I can remember [of] being drawn to pretty things, being drawn to my mother's jewellery box, wanting to skip with the girls in kindergarten and public school. I learned to be aggressive playing soccer, but I really didn't like it. If I had had my choice, I would have hung out with the girls and I would have played with pretty things. Those feelings never left as I grew older, but I suppressed them by becoming so determined that I was going to live a very clean-cut banker life and prove that I could be the perfect spouse, the perfect parent, the perfect corporate leader. But the feelings were always there; I just kept squishing them down. I think they're all related to this sense that you've got to fit into a box, and that sense of fitting into a box starts to get formed very early in life.
>
> But when you get older and your children get older, and your marriage matures and your career matures, it's hard to sustain that level of intensity that keeps things suppressed. As I got older, it started to boil over.

Katie's life changed when she was about fifty years old. By that point, she'd been working for her company for over thirty years, making her way to the top of a traditionally male-dominated profession and ticking all the boxes we normally associate with "success." And yet something was missing. Something major. The revelation about what that "something" was came during a visit with her daughter.

KD: I walked into my daughter's university dorm in September or August of 2016, and I saw a poster of somebody assigned male at birth wearing a silk blouse and pearls and full of joy, and the narrative on the poster said, "Embrace gender variance." And it stopped me dead in my tracks, and I thought, "Oh my goodness, could the world become so open that I could be me, the whole me?"

And then, in December of 2016, I'm in a barbershop, and there's a *National Geographic* on the coffee table in the waiting room titled "Gender Revolution," and I grab it. I did not know, Sophie, what gender was, but I was consumed by it, by these stories of countless young people expressing their true gender. I still didn't understand it, but it captivated me. It was speaking to me at a very near conscious or subconscious level.

I followed Caitlyn Jenner's story—and I do not relate to Caitlyn Jenner as a person; we're very different people—but it captivated me. I finally asked a dear friend from the LGBT community, "What the heck is going on with Caitlyn Jenner? Is this just another reality TV show?" And they told me about how she struggled with these feminine or female feelings her whole life. And how she poured herself into her career, into sports, to be busy and to be perfect, to suppress this part of her, but she couldn't outrun it and she had to face it.

SG: So one day you filmed a video and you explained what you were going through?

KD: I did, but the thought of not being able to preserve my career was causing me enormous distress. The video was about keeping my job so that I could finish putting my kids through university and save enough money so I could retire someday reasonably decently. And when I shared my personal journey and experience with the senior executive of the bank, I said, "I don't know how I'm going to do this, but I will find the strength to do this in my job."

In the video, the old version of me explained what I was going through. I showed a picture of my true self [as

Katherine]—a gorgeous picture, by the way. I explained my story with the greatest level of vulnerability and authenticity of the fact that I had struggled with anxiety and these feelings for my entire life, and that I could no longer outrun those feelings. And that when I returned in person to the office, I would be known as Katie.

SG: Incredible. How long were you away from the office?

KD: I worked remotely for two months. I had a little bit of surgery. I needed to spend time with my family. I needed to buy a new wardrobe. I needed to be ready to show up in my job with confidence and with credibility.

And what happened after the release of my video was the most profound experience of my life. I received hundreds—and now, three years later, thousands—of emails from countless colleagues and people in the broader community and from around the world. And the feedback fit into different categories: "Oh my goodness, you are incredible. We cannot get over your courage and your bravery." And I will go to my deathbed saying, "I do not know what you mean by *brave*," because I think heroes are brave, and all I did was fight to save myself, which is, I guess, what *bravery* really means. The second comment I got was "You're going to save lives," because I was such a visible senior leader. I have not found another leader in the world that has come out in front of twenty-five thousand employees in the division of the company that they lead.

On the negative side, somebody in my personal life sent around conversion therapy information to people that I love. And it was traumatizing to know that somebody I cared for and trusted was promoting this idea of converting me, when I darn well knew that any attempt, at this point in my life, to convert or suppress my true self would have probably resulted in suicide.

So, when I came out and shared my vulnerability, countless people trusted me enough to share their human stories and struggles, whether it was women, men that had suffered childhood trauma, people from the East Indian community, the Indigenous community, etc. And what I realized as a human, but even more so as a senior corporate and business leader, was the level of fear and anxiety and hurt that so many people carry around with them, regardless of what their story is. And how, like me, those people hold back part of their creativity, part of their uniqueness, because they're afraid of being outed; they're afraid of being judged or rejected by their company or the world. And what I realized is how much human potential society and our organizations or businesses miss out on because of this fear of not being perfect, of not fitting into a norm.

To see it so clearly, through my coming out, has been the single most transformative aspect of my life as a human being, but also in my profession as a corporate leader, and it has forever changed me. The world calls it a coming-out process, but it's really a journey of letting others into your personal life and truth. Sharing yourself with others is a gift, not an obligation. I look forward to the day when everyone can be their unique and beautiful self.

It's complex to go through a gender-affirming process. As I speak publicly about it now, I don't really care for the word *transgender*, because I did not transition my gender; I affirmed my gender. I am a woman, with gender-affirming experience— experience and insight that I consider a privilege.

SG: Would you agree that facing and telling your truth can be a miraculous revelation?

KD: For sure. You can't outrun your truth. You either reconcile with your truth along the way, or you reconcile with it on your deathbed. It will haunt you more and more as you get older, and show up in forms of illness, mental health issues, etc. I was convinced that I was going to be judged and rejected by the world, and that I would hurt my children and I would hurt my spouse. And like 80 to 90 percent of my community, I came very close to taking my life. And then a dear friend helped me realize that I would have hurt my children even more had I taken my life. And so, at that point, I wrote a letter of intention to myself to find the strength. And because I'm Canadian and it's a good country where my human rights are protected, and because I worked for a great company and because I had advisors and people around me to love me and support me, I told myself that I could do it as well or better than any human being has ever done it before.

SG: And how are you feeling these days?

KD: I'm at a point where, when I look in the mirror in the morning and I recognize the woman I see, I love her, and I'm at peace with who I am. As much as I love myself, like most people, I still have moments of high stress or anxiety where I feel guilt or shame or fear of being judged and rejected. Feeling like you are in the minority can be hard for anyone. I try to take care of myself. I believe in meditation and mindfulness as mechanisms to cope with and release fear and anxiety but, ultimately, to connect with your inner child and your true self. It's about authenticity. It's about living your truth and being truth in the world.

SG: I stand with you. We stand with you. But more than that, we're skipping with you!

KD: I can't wait to skip with you, too!

In late 2022, Katie took the next step in her journey and retired from the company she loved deeply. "Saying goodbye to the thousands of colleagues I worked with and who had embraced me was an incredibly painful experience," she said. "I wanted to move on young enough to be able to build a whole other career as Katie and only Katie. I feel blessed that I get to live another lifetime as all of me."

More than thirty years ago, when I was a teenager, no one talked about gender affirmation. It would have been very difficult to imagine bankers or CEOs living the transformational story Katie has lived. In so many ways, the winding road to finding your sense of purpose is more about the journey than the destination. If only I'd known this when I was a teenager! But then again, I doubt I would have had the patience for the process. There are some things you just need to grow into.

Fumbling toward Purpose (More than Once)

While in university, I was still struggling with my eating disorder, and I had no real idea of where I was headed. I had passion, interests, and talents, but the "never enough" note kept sounding in my head. My brain had taught me that I had to be perfect in order to keep my dad close and my mother happy. I'd convinced myself it was the only way we could all remain a unit. Without them, I wouldn't be just an only child; I'd be alone. Does that sound like a childish thought for a teenager to have? If only I'd had a choice in the matter. This was my hard-wiring at work, though I didn't know that yet.

Early on, my parents encouraged me to get some work experience to develop my sense of responsibility. It's a pattern I've followed with my own kids as well, encouraging Xavier and Ella-Grace to take on odd jobs and babysitting by their early teens. My early work opportunities taught me discipline and responsibility, and gave me a sense of accomplishment. I trust they will do the same for Xav and Ella.

I got my first summer job when I was fourteen. I worked the fifth hole "pit-stop cabin" of the St-Donat golf club in Lanaudière, Quebec, where I sold chocolate bars and cans of soda to mostly middle-aged male golfers. I kept a broom close by, because mice would come visit, too. I did my job very well, offered good customer service, and soon ended up working at the snack bar at the start of the course, which I enjoyed.

I had my first taste of stage performance (aside from ballet recitals) in Saint-Donat that summer as well. The youth community organized a talent show, and I was invited to join in. Apparently, my passion for gender-equality issues was already taking root: wearing ripped jeans

114

and a T-shirt, I danced and lip-synched along to "Woman's Work" by Tina Arena. I laugh now thinking about it. What did I know then about a woman's work? And yet, somehow, I'd picked up enough from the women in my life to allow the lyrics to resonate.

As time went by, jobs and opportunities came with a little more responsibility. I did a summer stint in the archives at my dad's office in downtown Montreal, mostly filing and clerical work. I was happy enough for the experience, but found the work so boring I promised myself I'd never do it again.

During university, I landed a job as a salesperson at Holt Renfrew in the Rockland shopping centre. Working during the school semester and on weekends while my friends were out and about wasn't always fun, but I loved sales, especially the contact with clients, and I had a passion for fashion, beauty, and design. I guess I made a good impression, because the general manager sat me down in his office a couple of months into it and said, "Sophie, I see a lot of people come in and out of here, and you've got natural talent. You're a hard worker and you have a lot to look forward to." Our paths crossed again a decade later, when I was working as a personal shopper at Holt's downtown location, and to this day I get the occasional supportive email from that same boss, and it always brings a smile to my face.

Apart from the sales experience I was gaining, I was definitely still "green" as far as the job market went. I finally moved out of my parents' home and found an apartment close by, where I lived with a small parakeet named Fiji, who loved taking showers, and a rabbit named Polka, who nibbled on the hems of my boyfriend's jeans and many of the cords in the house.

Fresh out of university, I applied to work at a small and relatively new advertising firm called Diesel Marketing. Their office on Avenue du Parc was an open-style loft, with work stations and a pool table. I knew nothing about the advertising world but was determined to look the part. The day of the interview, I dressed in a tailored suit and tie, and styled my then very short hair in an homage to Sharon Stone and Meg Ryan. I met with one of the founders, who was about ten years older than I was. We spoke for a full hour, and I guess he could sense my good social skills and can-do attitude, because I got a call later that week telling me I'd landed a job answering the phones and assisting the president in his daily tasks. I had a BA in communications, so it wasn't exactly my dream job, but I kept my head down and went for it. I met incredibly creative, witty, talented, and hard-working people there— bright entrepreneurs who were taking risks. It really felt like we were part of a fun team ready to take over the industry with our out-of-the-box approach to branding and advertising.

I soon became an account manager for big clients, and the team sent me on the road to try to bring in new business. I wasn't really prepared for it and made some rookie mistakes, but I wasn't going to back down from the challenge or the opportunity. I presented well, but on one occasion, the director of a well-known Quebec lingerie company told me (in a very kind way) to go back and do some more homework. Ouch. I was learning, all right. And I kept at it. I managed clients and accounts; performed voice-overs and posed for some crazy ads; toured ski stations for fondue tasting and branding exercises; joined in on magazine shoots, at recording studios, and on television ad sets—the list goes on.

I was doing well for a while and then, all of a sudden, I felt aimless again. I still didn't know what I wanted to do with my life. I was good at my job, but not quite good enough. I was living with my boyfriend at the time, and things weren't quite right with him either. No matter where I looked, I couldn't find a true sense of meaning and contribution. Perhaps not surprisingly, my bulimia episodes kicked in again. I was paying less attention at work, and it showed. One day, the president called me in for a meeting. He asked how I was doing and then let me know that they were (understandably) disappointed in my work. I couldn't hold it in anymore. I told my boss that I suffered from an eating disorder and that I was feeling lost. He was direct in telling me that things had to change, but he also showed warmth and compassion. I will never forget that moment. Speaking my truth had not cost me my job, and more than twenty years later, that same boss who'd believed in

116

me when I was fresh out of university asked me to speak at Canada's biggest conference on creativity: C2 Montreal.

I eventually left that job for a stint in public relations, and then landed work at *Les Ailes de la Mode* magazine. I sold advertising pages to some of their suppliers and met interesting creatives in the world of marketing, fashion, and sales. I enjoyed nourishing all those relationships, as well as the written work that the job required. I knew I was a talented communicator, and I also knew that I loved the entertainment world. So, after years of hopping between the sales, advertising, and public relations worlds, and feeling a bit like a butterfly who hadn't yet found the right flower to land on, I applied to a well-respected television and radio school in Montreal called Promedia. I got in, and my journey there was life-affirming. The comments I received from my teachers and fellow students were encouraging and confirmed my passion to work and prosper in the industry.

I was living alone in a one-bedroom apartment at that time, and I couldn't afford to be jobless. The freelance nature of work in my newly chosen field was hard to manage. I knocked on some doors and, through a close friend's connections, got an opportunity to work as a ticker writer at TVA's continuing news channel, LCN. You know those lines of news that appear on the bottom of your screen—what we call "chyrons" today? Well, I was working away at a computer in a tiny cubicle, mostly on night shifts, writing those words. Lacking experience, I made a couple of factual mistakes that almost cost me my job. I definitely cried in the bathroom once or twice, wondering if I was completely out of my league, but I kept at it.

Months later, there was a casting call for a Quebec cultural reporter at LCN. To my delight, I got the job. In the summer, I took on extra stints in early-morning radio (waking up at four a.m. to be in the studio for five or six), and I occasionally filled in as a co-host on the province's most-watched morning show, *Salut Bonjour*, staying in Quebec City for a couple of weeks at a time. I also took theatre classes with a well-known actor and coach in Montreal named Danielle Fichaud, which I really enjoyed.

For several years, I continued to do freelance work in television and radio. I hosted golf tournaments where half the crowd was drunk and rowdy, and peewee hockey playoffs, where I sometimes forgot to pass the microphone to the guest I was interviewing. I made mistakes during live conversations while trying to look like I wasn't wearing an earpiece (and yet still listening to the control room and reading off a teleprompter). I was learning big-time, and there were plenty of occasions when I hit walls and had to make myself get back up. Eventually, I found a good agent to represent me. One thing led to another, and I started hosting shows on arts and technology, extreme sports, and wildlife. I also began volunteering and got involved with organizations such as BACA (Boulimie, Anorexie, Comportements Alimentaires) and Shield of Athena, which is a nonprofit organization for victims of family violence. Only then did I feel I'd found my true calling. Working in television and radio *and* being able to give back was very fulfilling. I simply loved it. Finally, I felt I was offering myself to the world in a way that could make a difference. And I wanted to make a big one. As years went by, I had the privilege of working as an interviewer in both French and English Canada. I sat down with fascinating personalities who also wanted to have a positive impact in people's lives. In 2023, as I was sharing dinner with one of my former bosses, with whom I'd formed a great friendship over time, he reminded me of how adamant I was about sharing positive and impactful stories when we first met during my hiring process almost two decades earlier. This desire allowed me to conduct conversations with people from all walks of life, such as Malala Yousafzai, Justin Timberlake, Dan Aykroyd, Hillary and Chelsea Clinton, Brad Pitt, and many more.

Redefining Success

Now that I look back, I realize that my love for the stage, my innate curiosity for learning and teaching, as well as my attraction to (and love-hate relationship with) retail and fashion had been with me for most of my life. It makes sense now that I've found fulfillment in working as a yoga teacher and a public speaker, and that being on a stage feels like home. A part of me wishes I could have figured out earlier what really makes me tick, but all those experiences and the people I met along the way showed me my path, whether it was intentional or not.

What feels much less like home is the narrow concept of success that we have all grown up with. Society says that success is recognition and accumulation of wealth. I say it's contribution and interconnectedness.

One expression that has always been overused in relation to career achievement is "self-made." I believe that every single person you meet has a role to play in your development, no matter if the encounter is positive or negative. The idea that we are the sole creator of our own success story creates a distorted view of reality. It's too narrow, too self-centred. And how likely are we to want to give back, or to pay it forward, if we don't feel we owe at least a little bit of who we are to each other? "People is business and business is people!" was my dad's favourite line. There is truth to this, and more and more these days, we are hearing from people who are figuring this out—people who are redefining success, tapping into their own passions and sense of purpose, and changing the world for the better.

Jake Karls is one of those people. I met him in 2022, and our conversation left me with a deep sense of hope for our younger generations. Jake, who made *Forbes* magazine's "30 under 30" list in 2023, is the co-founder of the "functional chocolate bar" company Mid-Day Squares, and his purpose in life is to make people feel deeply, to spread good energy, and to show the world that you can win by being yourself, unapologetically, every day. I wanted to hear more about his unique and wholly authentic success story.

Sophie Grégoire: You're a business leader and entrepreneur, but people are taken aback when they meet you. They think,

"Whoa, he's not the typical 'man in a suit,' is he?" How do you react to that?

Jake Karls: I'm twenty-nine years old, and when I started this business, I was twenty-five, so I was really, really young. And most people doubted me at the beginning and still do. I would show up in a beach shirt, because sometimes that's who I am, and I felt the judgment; I felt that this was something they didn't want to see. And that really irritated me.

I'm just trying to be me, in my life. And when I started to really embrace that and stop fearing the judgment and thinking about what others think, my mind went free. Because the second I try to be somebody else—or I go into the "standard" box, the rigidity—that's when I'm going to start to fail, because then I can't be the best version of myself. There'll be moments of difficulty where I really doubt myself, but I can't let somebody else make me feel that way, because that feeling is a mental prison, and I hate it.

SG: You talk about doubt. What did that feel like for you?

JK: I've gone through all of the emotions. Guilt: Am I doing what I'm supposed to be doing in life? Am I being the person I'm supposed to be? Ashamed, in the sense of, am I embarrassing myself by dancing with everyone, making people laugh? Am I looked at as a class clown? At times during this journey, I felt very depressed and very sad and alone.

I never did really well academically in school, so I always had this insecurity that I was unable to write; I was unable to do public speaking. I never got good at it because I have something called dyspraxia—which is all about fine motor skills—and didn't know until I was twenty-three years old. So, for me, handwriting is extremely difficult. Doing up buttons on a shirt is very difficult. Tying my shoes takes me so long. It's just my brain's not processing it. I grew up playing hockey, and in the locker rooms, everyone's parents would do their skates up to a certain point. But my mom had to continue coming even when I was a teenager. That insecurity carried through till I was an adult, and I always felt like, "I'm not good enough." It took a lot of therapy and work to understand that about myself.

SG: Do you think that your generation, your fellow millennials, are suffering emotionally?

JK: I feel like they aren't breaking through. Growing up, they were told, "You need to get a job here; you need to do this; you need to do that," and that's what stuck to them. So what I'm noticing now is this unhappiness or lack of fulfillment, where they have not achieved what they truly want to achieve; their purpose has not been met. My mission is to show people—being a plumber, flying planes, starting a chocolate company, going into journalism, whatever it is—that if you follow your gut and you can withstand the pressure of what people are going to say around you or what social media is going to say, then you can succeed. But you need to be able to withstand that deep pressure.

You need to withstand the deep pressure, know how to sit with the pain—that's some pretty amazing advice for life, but when you apply it to the business world, it takes on a different dimension. Imagine if more corporations were tuned in to the kinds of things Jake is talking about: encouraging employees to embrace their authentic selves and find their purpose, or tap into their true potential. When I asked Jake about what he'd learned about himself in therapy and how he applied that knowledge to his work as an entrepreneur, he told me a great story:

JK: My business partners are my sister and my brother-in-law. They said to me, when we started the business, "Hey, if you want to be the third partner, you need to accept that we are going to see a therapist once a week, mandatory, good or bad times, so we can work on our communication and on under-standing each other and being empathetic and learning how to communicate at a very high level."

And I kind of felt embarrassed, Sophie, to go to therapy at the time. I was like, "This is weird; I don't need it," and they're like, "Well, if you don't commit to it, then you can't join as a third partner." I went to the first session and it was like taking bullets, I swear to you. I felt like my ego just got completely shot. And then, finally, after three, four, five, six sessions, I started to embrace therapy. I was like, oh my god, this is a place where I could actually develop myself as a human. It allows you to gain perspective.

I've become so much more empathetic in my life. I listen first; I don't talk first now. I've learned that when someone's attacking me, it doesn't mean that it's coming from a place of hate. They might be going through something, and understanding that and having a space for them is a whole other game.

So, when you ask what therapy does, it helps me to become more secure in myself, where I could actually be wrong and I'm okay with being wrong. And I'm okay that you were right and I'm cheering you on for that. And I think that's how we succeed going forward in any type of relationship, friendship, or business partnership.

SG: On a last note, I think it is our birthright as human beings to have an opportunity to develop a sense of purpose. What do you think is the greatest gift you can give somebody to develop that sense of purpose?

JK: Start putting yourself in uncomfortable scenarios. Do something that you haven't done before. Because the moment you step into the uncomfortable, you start to experience something you've never experienced. You might meet somebody. You never know what that conversation is going to lead to, what door that might open, and what friendship that might build. And as soon as you start doing it consistently, I can guarantee you the world's your oyster.

Leading (and Loving) Yourself

Let's keep things straight here: finding your passions and purpose and defining your sense of self is not a linear process. But when you make wise decisions regarding how you give to yourself and contribute to this world, in tiny or big ways, things get so much easier. "Purpose is spirit seeking expression," writes author Kevin Cashman.

I have a dear friend who knows this from personal experience. You may know Mark Tewksbury as the Olympian who dominated in the pool at the Seoul and Barcelona Olympics, bringing home gold, silver, and bronze medals for Canada. Almost twenty years ago, Mark came out as Canada's first openly gay sports star, and has been a leader and mentor in the global LGBTQ+ human rights movement ever since. He has been chair of Special Olympics Canada, a vice president of the Canadian Olympic Committee, and co-founder of Great Traits, a leadership training and development company.

Despite his long list of accomplishments, Mark hasn't always had an easy path. Speaking about his decision to come out, he told me, "I went through a period of my life where I was on the floor, fetal position, so depressed, so sick. And it was because, in my mind, the fact that I was gay meant I was bad, or I was wrong or something. And so I just couldn't function. That thought took over."

Mark knew he had to get help, but it was hard to take those first steps. "My ego was telling me, 'I'm an Olympic champion; I don't need to talk to somebody.' But I did. I went back to university; I studied sexual and gender politics. I started to become educated, found a language. And once I found a language, all of a sudden, my perception of what my reality was started to change."

We spoke more about his work in development and training, and what it can teach all of us about the importance of living an authentic life.

Sophie Grégoire: It sounds like what broke you also built you. What are you teaching others about leadership and having emotional agency over ourselves?

Mark Tewksbury: We look at it from three different perspectives. First is leading yourself—those are the achiever traits—how to set goals, how to hold yourself accountable, how to persevere, how to build a support team, how to be innovative. The second level is what we call leadership traits. They build on the same ideas that are in the achiever but with a different point of view. Many people are excellent at their job, and then they get promoted as a super-achiever into a leadership position, and it's something totally different. Leadership is no longer about being the best and a super-achiever; it's about facilitating ten people below you to be better than you were. And then comes legacy.

SG: So, in order to lead—either ourselves or others—we must have more self-awareness?

MT: Yes. I'll give you a quick example: I was called in to speak to the Vancouver 2010 Olympic team right before the opening ceremony. They'd had a death on the luge track that morning, so we started the pep rally with a moment of silence. I had this really powerful FDR, Nelson Mandela-type speech prepared, but I saw that the team was going to just crumble if I gave that speech. They're feeling so much grief, they're not sure how to be.

If you told me, "Mark, you're going to do stand-up comedy to the Vancouver 2010 team," I'd have said, "Never." But I went up there and shared all the things that ever went wrong in my career, and I got everyone laughing. And that was what was needed in that moment.

A great leader needs super-awareness, because you've got to figure out what this person or this situation needs that's best for them. And it might be something in your arsenal that you haven't used for twenty years, but it's the right thing in this moment.

SG: Experts say that it takes two minutes, when you're stuck on negative thoughts, to bring your attention to something else, and whoop, you'll kind of forget about your negative thoughts. Can you imagine what we could do with three minutes, fifteen minutes, an hour per day, or whatever life allows you to have? We can change our brains.

MT: It all boils down to awareness and self-reflection. And I think some people are so reactionary, they're not even stopping to realize, "Oh my god, I'm going through this whole day from a place of doubt or fear or whatever it is." You have to be aware enough to take the two minutes to start to change the way your brain is working.

SG: Does a leader have to genuinely like themselves in order to lead others?

MT: That's a really interesting question. I think so, because there's this energy and synergy that we can't see with the eye. If that is true, then your thoughts are the start of igniting the energy that you have. And so, if you're really negative and hate yourself, you're just not going to be able to access your full potential. Even worse, it's going to be hard not to eventually leak that onto the people you're leading, without even knowing it.

SG: Do you like yourself?

MT: I love myself.

What a perfect note to end on, because we'll be talking a whole lot about love in the next chapter. And as we'll learn from the incredible experts we meet there, developing a good sense of self—like Katie, and Jake, and Mark, and so many of us have by following our own winding roads—is vitally important when it comes to connecting healthily with others, whether in platonic or romantic relationships. In the next chapter, we'll discover life-changing ways to deepen your most cherished bonds and learn how to keep them strong, even in times of struggle. Let's rock this love boat.

What Makes You Light Up?

At some point or another, we all struggle to discover our passions and purpose—the things that make us light up. I spent years trying different jobs before I figured out the kind of work that nourishes my heart and soul, and makes me feel as if I am contributing.

On the website BetterUp, Maggie Wooll writes that "just thinking about 'purpose and passion' can be paralyzing." Thankfully, Wooll goes on to pose a series of questions we can ask ourselves if we're still struggling to put the pieces together, or if we just want to check in on this issue that is so important to our mental health and well-being. Grab a notebook or journal and see where this exercise takes you:

- What keeps me coming back to learn more, no matter how much I already know?
- What activities bring me joy and/or excitement and keep me so engaged that I lose track of time?
- What are my skills, talents, and strengths? What am I good at?
- What issues do I care about, and why do I care about them?

Once you've answered these questions, you can start to connect your passions and purpose in meaningful ways. Do the passions you had at other points in your life have anything in common with the things that bring you joy now? Pay attention to the common threads that may be emerging, because they may be pointing toward your purpose.

Next, consider the different ways you spend your time. Do they align with your passions?

Finally, open yourself up to new opportunities that use your skills and tap into the things that bring you joy. From blogging to building a community garden, for example, there are as many options out there as there are people trying to seize them.

Tapping into your passion and purpose isn't a "one and done" proposition. We are constantly changing and growing, so the things that bring joy and meaning to our lives will change, too. Make a promise to yourself to revisit these questions from time to time, especially if you find yourself feeling stuck or uninspired.

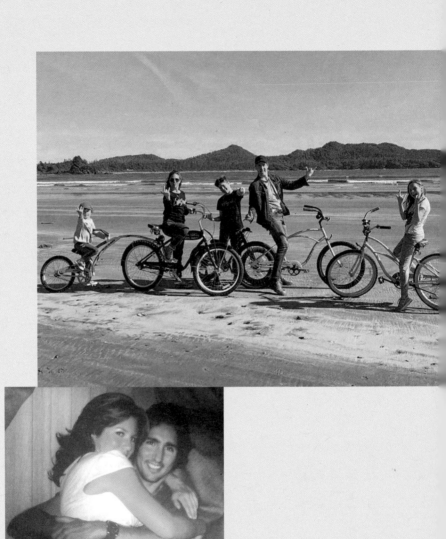

5

The Heart of the Matter

A Whole Lot about Love

For small creatures such as we the vastness of
the universe is bearable only through love.

CARL SAGAN

For as long as I can remember, I've always felt "in love"—in love with life, nature, animals, music, movement, dance, breathing, the wind in my hair, the way light enters a window, strangers smiling at each other, a wrinkly face filled with history, the depth and space of time, and all of life's mystery. When I get to offer love, I feel more alive than ever. Sometimes I can't believe I get to be human, and I often think about the infinitesimally small odds of your soul being born into this world. My true nature wants to seek connection. So does yours. Our brains are wired for it in order to survive, and no matter the form of love—romantic, platonic, familial—it can affect our physical and

It is possible to speak with our heart directly. Most ancient cultures know this. We can actually converse with our heart as if it were a good friend. In modern life we have become so busy with our daily affairs and thoughts that we have lost this essential art to converse with our heart.

JACK KORNFIELD

psychological well-being. In this chapter, we're going to focus primarily on romantic love in all its complexity.

Did you know that quality relationships and love can be a buffer against stress? The brain areas associated with reward and pleasure are at play as a relationship grows. And when we feel a deep sense of peace, contentment, and calm with our loved one, it can help alleviate physical pain and build more compassion, better creativity, and better memory. Love can help us foster safer behaviours and reduce worry and nervousness. A healthy relational support system can even lower the chances of developing depression or other forms of mental illness.

You know that natural high you can feel when you've spent time in connection with someone you love? That feeling is stored in the brain, and just thinking about that special person or moment can bring joy and alleviate negative thoughts. But because there is a flip side to every coin, love can also feel like an addiction. And just like addictive drugs, love can ignite our pleasure centres and result in mood swings, cravings, emotional dependence, and more.

I wanted to share some of these findings with you (there are so many studies on the impacts of love on the brain, body, and mood) because I think it's important to understand that our core need for human contact and deep presence, as well as secure and validating relationships, is not capricious or narcissistic. While many experts agree that we can live full lives without a primary intimate relationship or sex, touch (without sex) is still important. Whether from a

SOPHIE GRÉGOIRE TRUDEAU

friend, a pet, or a caregiver, touch calms our nervous system. Without it, we can become irritable and even angry or depressed. We are not asking for too much when we want our partners or close friends to show up for us as we show up for them. But as we all know, long-term relationships are not easy to manage. In order to nourish and sustain relationships, we must constantly adapt to change and to how both we and the other person evolve through time and experience. This is just one reason why we must be willing to examine ourselves and our interpersonal dynamics: doing so helps our relationships to be more peaceful and loving.

I once asked my teenage son what he thought the rhythm of love is. To my amazement, he didn't roll his eyes and leave the room. Instead, he remained silently thoughtful for a time, and then he said, "Slow?" After I recovered from my shock, I said, "Well, Xav, you pretty much have the secret of life summed up in one word!" No one can truly feel safe and loved without slowing down. When you slow down, if you feel secure enough to do so, you create the conditions necessary to connect with yourself and others in a truthful way. The rhythm of indifference is fast; it doesn't allow for this introspection. But Xavier was right: the rhythm of love *is* slow.

You don't need to take my word for it—or Xav's! The next time you hug someone you feel close to, try to slow that hug down. Hold it for at least thirty seconds. Do you feel that light elation and release? Sometimes I'll ask my kids for a thirty-second hug, and although they *do* roll their eyes at that, they've also been honest about how good it makes them feel.

True intimacy expresses itself in silence, in breath. In many ways, it imitates nature. When we love deeply and healthily, we do not feel rushed. We feel as if we can actually bend or extend time. We feel rested, at home, fulfilled. Maybe not 100 percent of the time—none of us is perfect, remember, and love isn't always easy. On the whole, though, love outweighs its obstacles.

But there are big questions lurking underneath all this talk about love, and the answers are so important to our relationships. Where do we learn how to love? How and when are we taught to nourish our relationships? Do we model ourselves after our parents' dynamics, or try to run miles away from what we witnessed as children? How is it that some of us seem to be better at relationships than others? The answer to this last and far from simple question is: self-awareness, vulnerability, creativity, and work.

Belgian-American psychotherapist and human relationship expert Esther Perel has suggested that thanks to our society's pretty puritan way of looking at couple dynamics, most of us would rather "kill" a relationship than question or change its structure. It's as if we've been taught that relationships either work or they don't. The way that usually plays out in our society is through marriage (defined as the "success" of a relationship) or divorce (the "failure"). But relationships aren't black or white—though we tend to categorize them that way, don't we? If only we could learn to slow down and understand ourselves better, and to trust in the other, we could build more enriching relationships. As Perel wrote in *Mating in Captivity: Unlocking Erotic Intelligence*, "The more we trust, the further we are able to venture." But in order to venture, we need to feed our emotional soil.

"What we nourish, we help grow. What we neglect becomes weaker." One of my favourite yoga and meditation teachers, Travis Eliot, said this during class one day. I believe these words to be true— whether what we are nourishing is a plant, our own body, or a relationship. The way we love is a deep revelation about ourselves.

Open communication, vulnerability, and honesty are paramount to a healthy dialogue. But in order for this to happen, we must feel secure. Our *brains* must feel secure. All too often, though, we carry emotional baggage into our relationships that prevents us from feeling this way. It goes back to that childhood bond of attachment we talked about in chapter 1, and how it plays out once we find ourselves in a relationship.

The Baggage We Bring

Justin and I had known each other as kids, but we reconnected when I was in my late twenties. There was a sense of tender familiarity in the air at the first rehearsal of the fundraising event we'd been asked to co-host. The night of the event, the vibe was definitely fun, outgoing, flirtatious, but that's as far as it went. I wrote him an email the next day saying it was great to have met again and to wish him the best of luck on his other projects. When it went unanswered, I was disappointed. We bumped into each other on the street later that year, and he asked for my number. I declined, telling him that if he really wanted it, he could find it. And so, when the phone rang one day when I was having lunch at a local café, I was a bit taken aback.

To make a long story short, we went for dinner in Montreal, and then ice cream, and then karaoke, and then back to his place. Right before he was going to drive me home in his rusty Bronco truck (which used to belong to his beloved late brother and smelled like moth-balls), the conversation turned to deeper topics, and he looked at me with such intense presence that I knew something special was going on. He said, "I'm thirty-one years old. I've been waiting for you for thirty-one years. Should we skip the girlfriend phase and start with fiancée?"

The rest, as they say, is history.

History, maybe, but not all smooth sailing. We met in 2003, he asked for my hand in 2004, and we married in 2005. But a few months before the wedding, my parents separated for the first time. When I learned of their decision, I was happy that they would each be getting a fresh start, but I think I was also in shock. Our trio had transformed into something unfamiliar. They were no longer a unit, so I felt like *we* were no longer a unit. And yet that unit was all I had ever known.

In the wake of my parents' announcement, I started having what I now recognize as panic attacks—dizzy spells that would strike completely out of the blue at work, home, and friends' houses, and even on the ski hill. I had no idea what was happening to me, but I did take steps to learn more about anxiety and how it could manifest. Around the same time, I'd also started going to therapy to figure out some of the deep worries and emotional patterns that weren't helping me to grow in my relationship with this man I was going to marry and build a family with. I was on a big learning curve. I'd chosen to understand more about myself so I could better interact with the people I loved most.

After a couple of sessions with a kind and brilliant therapist, I figured out that I had a little voice pattern inside me. It often said things like: "Not good enough. You're failing again. You can do more and better." My quest for perfectionism, which was rooted in guilt and also in shame, kept hurting me. It felt like a sharp hook wrapped around my neck—a constant emotional sting. With the help of therapy and a lot of work, I began to be able to see these negative defence mechanisms and emotional patterns as traits I could "observe" from a distance. I was learning more about them, and about how to intervene and change my way of thinking and feeling. One day during a session, I decided to turn that sharp metal hook into a bright-pink, feathery one—one that was more playful and felt like it tickled more than ripped my skin apart. And you know what? I think that mental technique helped me to befriend my negative thought process and learn how to navigate around it. And the relationships I hold dear are better, stronger, as a result.

I'm certainly not the first person to have gained knowledge and perspective about a relationship through therapy. Dr. John Grey can speak to that. Over the past three decades, he has helped thousands of couples save their marriages. In his internationally recognized and pioneering retreat program, John guides couples to communicate well, repair ruptures, overcome reactive cycles, and collaborate as a team. He regularly helps partners on the brink of divorce renew positive feelings and build solid, secure relationships to thrive as a couple. He's authored several self-help books, including *Five-Minute Relationship Repair*, that offer practical tools and principles for couples to overcome negative patterns and maximize shared happiness.

Artistic duo Raine Maida and Chantal Kreviazuk introduced me to John, who is featured in their insightful documentary on loving relationships, *I'm Going to Break Your Heart*. Originally a scholar, John switched to working with couples after a personal tragedy. "Within one year, my entire immediate family died. I had three deaths and I wasn't emotionally equipped to deal with it," he told me, explaining that the experience sent him looking for guidance on how to process his loss emotionally. "So I jumped over the fence into the realm of therapy, feelings—how do you process things, how do you work with trauma, how's all my childhood stuff coming up?"

When it comes to relationships, John says that most people don't start with these issues in mind, because at the beginning, everything feels so great. But he believes we *should* think about the past as we navigate the present, especially when it comes to love. And so, when I wanted to better understand why relationships can be so challenging, I reached out to Dr. Grey.

Sophie Grégoire: Why do we have such a difficult time navigating relationships?

Dr. John Grey: Well, I would say essentially because relationships are complex. And we lack—personally and probably, I would say, societally—sufficient models to embrace the complexity and translate that into things we can do, things we can say, ways we can communicate with each other that promote and foster lasting happiness.

SG: How do you help couples embrace that complexity?

JG: In the last twenty years, my model's shifting toward becoming better at interdependency—what I call a Love 3.0 model. The old "learn to love yourself first" is not a model for being a couple. That's a model for being an individual.

SG: With Love 3.0, you have to take care of two brains, not just one, right?

JG: That's the problem with relationships—it's called the two-brain problem. There's someone else over there, and inside their skull, there's a differently wired brain, and no matter how synched up it all feels in the beginning—and it's just magical and you finish each other's sentences, and you both like the same brand of crunchy peanut butter, isn't that amazing?—later down the road, you're going to find there's differences that start encroaching, different needs at the same time that are opposite, and that will be triggering. And as you become more and more important to each other as a couple, your attachment wiring is increasingly engaged—your brain wiring for being emotionally bonded with a significant other. This engages survival circuits, in that your original significant other was your parent.

SG: So you're saying we carry all of that baggage from our childhood into our adult relationships?

JG: It's all in your wiring. As adults, if you're in a strong, emotionally bonded relationship, you will trigger each other. And the way in which you get triggered is directed by the wiring that's in your brain. A lot of that wiring was created in the attachment period before the age of two. And more was built between two and fourteen. A lot was created in your teenage insecure years. A lot might have been created in a previous marriage or another significant relationship. So it's all in your brain. That wiring, as complex as it is, will be reflected in how you react, what you think about when reactions are happening. And it also pairs up with your specific partner. Different people will trigger each other in different ways.

This is such an important point that it's worth hitting pause on this fascinating conversation for a moment. John is telling us here that when it comes to relationships, past is always present. Whether it's how you were raised or the relational experiences you accumulated through living, it all impacts your present (for a peek into how your own past and experiences may be affecting your relationship present, check out the "Finding Your Attachment Style" quiz at the end of this chapter).

Dr. Grey is far from alone in this thinking. Terry Real is an internationally recognized family therapist, author, and teacher who is particularly known for his groundbreaking work on men and male psychology, as well as his work on gender and couples. In 1997, he published the bestseller *I Don't Want to Talk about It*, the first book ever written on the topic of male depression. His most recent work is another bestseller: *Us*. Like John Grey, he believes that what happened to us as children is always front and centre in our relationships, especially when situations crop up that can leave us feeling unsafe.

"Abraham Maslow said a met need is not a motivator," he told me. "If I'm not safe, all bets are off, I mean—food, water, sex, company, all that's fine, but if I'm going to die, that comes first. So the first order of business is [being] safe." He continued:

Terry Real: But what makes life tricky is that my autonomic nervous system can very easily say, "Terry, you're not safe," because of trauma. When, in fact, objectively, I am safe, but I don't know that I'm safe, because what's happening in the present is close enough to what happened to me as a little boy, that was not safe, that I get confused.

Trauma-triggering is a confusion. You don't remember trauma; you relive it. I'm not thinking I'm a seventy-two-year-old man remembering being beaten as a kid; I am that beaten kid in that moment. And then my adaptive child comes in to rescue that beaten kid and fight over and over and over and over again. I'm no longer the adult; I'm a four-year-old boy—that's what my body is feeling—I've got this towering six-foot-two father screaming at me, and I'm ready to punch somebody.

Powerful stuff, right? And it's echoed by Dr. Harville Hendrix and Dr. Helen LaKelly Hunt, partners in life and business (you may have seen Harville on *The Oprah Winfrey Show*). They are the co-creators of Imago Relationship Therapy and a social movement called Safe Conversations, and are internationally respected as therapists, educators, speakers, activists, and authors (their ten books, including the timeless classic *Getting the Love You Want*, have sold more than four million copies). They tell couples who are struggling or looking for a deeper connection to have empathy for one another, and to learn about each other's childhood experiences, wounds, and traumas. This is crucial, Helen told me, because of the way we can get triggered during tough discussions. "When I say something in a certain way to Harville," she said, "he's suddenly eight years old and he's mad. His mother treated him this way; his parents didn't notice him. He got triggered in his old wound. So two people need to spend time learning about a childhood challenge, and if a partner is upsetting them, they need to go, 'I wonder if that has to do with childhood?' And 'Can I be different from how his parents were that made him feel a certain way?'"

Knowing about this baggage we all carry is so important, but it's only half of the equation. The other half is knowing how to manage it—or even just accepting that it's an issue that needs to be addressed in order to have a happy, healthy, and secure relationship. As John Grey and I continued our conversation, he explained that failure to pay attention really isn't an option.

JG: Without course-correcting, this will get worse over time. So something might trigger a couple to a certain extent early in a relationship. You come back later and that same kind of thing is triggering much bigger reactions. Those upsets will be stored in the long-term wiring, and they will tend to amplify over time into negative generalizations about what to expect in this relationship. And out of those generalizations are our patterns of defence against that, but then our patterns trigger the other person even more. So it's a big circle where everybody's triggering each other, largely based on misperceptions in their own brains. The reactive behaviours that come out of

138

those get misperceived by the other party, and nobody knows what to do with any of that.

What they try to do never works. They try to explain it. You know, "I'm going to explain to my emotionally upset partner why she shouldn't be upset, and that's my best tool for repair. It backfires only about 100 percent of the time, so I'll try it again." But it's not the right kind of tool.

SG: What are the right tools, then?

JG: There are two things you really have to know how to do to manage this two-brain problem. You have to know how to repair upsets, because nobody's smart enough to prevent them 100 percent of the time. And you have to know how to do that emotionally, and therein is the rub.

The way I look at it is that people are generally trying to use left-brain tools to solve right-brain issues. It's not that they have bad intentions; they just don't have the tools. Left brain is more linear, cognitive—very complex speech patterns, ideas, theories, making meaning intellectually. Right brain is a parallel processing, non-linear, more emotional, relational body-based system. And that's where most of the triggering happens. Because most of what we're actually talking about when couples are having a problem is how they feel. Does it feel good or does it feel bad? Am I upset or am I happy? Do I feel connected in a positive way or am I apprehensive and insecure around my significant other? Couples need the tools to collaborate to get to win-win—which means both feel secure.

Getting to a Win-Win

Getting to win-win in a relationship sounds great, doesn't it? But how do we do it? How do we learn the right way to repair the hurts (big and small) and everyday grievances that are a feature of all relationships, regardless of form? As it turns out, Xavier was on the right track when he guessed that the rhythm of love is slow. When I asked John Grey about relationship repair, he affirmed that slow is exactly the right speed.

He asked me to think about talking a two-year-old down from a tantrum (it wasn't at all hard to remember those times). You go slow. You're attentive. You make contact; you touch them, hold them, maybe even look into their eyes. You speak slowly. He explained that all of this is also true for adults, if we want to get into that right-brain feeling centre. "The triggering is largely happening in that attachment wiring," he said, "and then our left-brain negative thoughts only amplify our upset."

So how, I wondered, do we learn to regulate that? This, too, goes back to our childhood experiences.

SG: Let's go back to the two-year-old having a tantrum. Say we're talking about a child whose parent slowed down, who gave them attention and physical care when they were angry or sad, and then waited until the child calmed down, and asked, "Are you okay?" And only when they felt sure that the child was okay would they say, "Now you can go back into the world." Would that child—grown up now—have a better regulatory system in a relationship?

JG: The research plainly shows that the more you get that kind of ideal distress relief co-regulation in childhood, the more your frontal brain is able to connect back into your survival-alarm brain and calm that amygdala down to self-regulate and keep your brain more steady. The analogy, roughly, is like having brakes on the car to balance with the accelerator. The fight-flight system is like an accelerator—it puts more gas in the system, and you go faster and faster and faster. Having brakes is the self-regulating system that will slow you down. And the better brakes you have probably the quicker you can start resolving triggering and stay steady in order to engage in that very complicated task of repair.

SG: What would you tell most couples when they face a conflict? What are, let's say, the three most important steps we can take to manage this situation?

JG: I use the acronym CPR—catch, pause, repair. In medicine, it's cardiopulmonary resuscitation. Back when I started thirty years ago, I had the CP part pretty well mapped out—catch and pause; take a time out; centre yourself. When you're getting triggered, you don't have the equipment in your brain to solve the problem. It's actually being turned off by the survival system—which is not what you need. You need your higher brain to solve the triggering, so you need to take the time out, get your higher brain back to calm, regulate yourself, and then come back.

But that's just CP. It's obviously insufficient for the whole medical analogy. You don't just stand around saying, "The patient is having a cardiopulmonary event" and then walk away, satisfied that you know what it is. No, you need resuscitation. And the R is the most important thing in relationships, too: catch, pause, and *repair*. Emotional repair is where it's at. And it's very valuable for a number of reasons. The first and most obvious is it helps you deal with the immediate upset and not only get over it but actually get reconnected in a positive, healing way.

SG: What does a good repair look like?

JG: You have to be able to directly address the real insecurities that are getting throttled up and ringing the brain's survival alarm. You have to know how to speak to those. How do you really calm the other person down and make them feel secure with you? This is essential and it's a very simple process, but most people are not doing it well.

SG: In our society, we have not been taught—like math is taught or French is taught or language is taught—how to repair a conflict between two human beings.

JG: Correct. We don't even get taught in therapy how to do it, never mind school. For instance, here's something everybody

141

tries to do: A couple's upset; they want to try to repair it in the moment. Let's say they're enlightened. They have a time-out word. They pause. They come back. They get back into the same issue again. Both of them need a repair. But neither one is able to deliver it when they're both trying to go for it at once. What I've found is, you have to go one way at a time. Everybody should be repaired, needs to be repaired, but there has to be a repairer and a repairee.

SG: How important is deep listening in conflict resolution?

JG: Deep listening is extremely important, but then deep speaking is what matches it. You can't do deep listening if all you're hearing is a bunch of surface-level complaints and criticisms. I would submit you're not able to listen deeply unless you can speak deeply. What that means, specifically, is getting underneath the content issue you think you're upset by into the actual emotional realm underneath.

SG: So take the leap of being vulnerable.

JG: Yeah, that's it. Vulnerability is really the key. Without it, you're just going to stay on the surface, arguing over things. We have to be able to be comfortable, or get more comfortable, or help each other become more comfortable being vulnerable, because that's the only way we can actually talk about what's really going on.

Now we're getting somewhere. Vulnerability is one of the keys to relationship repair, but being vulnerable is hard, especially when we're feeling emotionally bruised. It makes sense, then, that learning how to talk to and interact with our partner to support vulnerability is an important first step. Here again, our attachment styles come into play. John Grey often uses popular nicknames for the two insecure attachment styles: "island" for the avoidant, and "wave" for the anxious, ambivalent, preoccupied, anger-resistant. Knowing whether you're a wave or an island—and also knowing what your partner is—can make a big difference when you're in the middle of a

142

disagreement. John has a quiz that can help us figure this out (it's at the end of this section, on page 147).

Islands, as you might guess, didn't receive very much distress relief in childhood, and so they've learned how to take care of their own stress. "They will show up in relationships as adults with a kind of pride in their independence," John Grey explained. "They're not needy emotionally like other people are. They can just go off and take care of themselves. They don't really like talking about feelings. It can easily overwhelm them because they don't have much practice in it. They will tend to just want to go off and be on their own and calm down. And then come back and everybody should be happy."

Waves did get some attention and distress relief as kids, so they know it exists. But it maybe wasn't always there when they needed it. Maybe their parents had to work a lot; maybe the parents themselves became upset easily; or maybe there was some role reversal at work, and the child ended up having to take care of the parents. It doesn't really matter what created the wave attachment style; the outcome is the same. As John explains, "The basic idea is, when waves get upset, they tend to want to go *toward* the other and get relief, and yet there's this whole history of inconsistency in their past, so the way they try to do it will tend to overwhelm. They'll tend to emote more, express more. And so quite often, couples will find themselves in a dilemma that resembles an island/wave, pursuer/withdrawer reactive cycle. And that will happen even if they're both waves, or both islands. The one who's more of an island will turn the other into more of a wave, in general."

No wonder we so often make a mess of conflict resolution. With all of our emotional baggage and communication-style issues in the mix, talking through a disagreement with our partner can feel like walking through a minefield. You take tentative steps, fully expecting something to explode. It can also feel profoundly draining for one or both partners. But it doesn't have to be this way. We can learn how to communicate better, with respect and humility and, above all else, love. I checked in with Harville Hendrix and Helen LaKelly

Hunt about this. Not only have they made thirty years of their relationship work, but they also designed a communication system specifically for fostering understanding, empathy, and connection. Here's how it works:

- The partners agree on one topic of conversation. One partner speaks at a time and chooses to be either the Sender or Receiver.
- When the Sender speaks, they use "I" statements. They try not to blame, label, mind-read, or say "you always" or "you never," and they stay focused on the topic at hand. They keep their tone of voice, posture, and gestures non-threatening and non-accusatory, and they pause now and again to let the Receiver respond.
- The Receiver's response includes three steps. First, when the Sender pauses, the Receiver repeats back—or *mirrors*—what they heard, without analysis or critiques. The Receiver asks if anything was missed and if there is more the Sender wishes to say. Second, if the Sender is finished, the Receiver *validates* what they heard and how it makes sense. If anything didn't make sense, they ask for further clarification. Third, the Receiver *empathizes*, guessing what the Sender might be feeling regarding their issue (if the Sender already said how they feel, the Receiver can simply mirror this back once more).
- When the Sender is finished and the Receiver has mirrored, validated, and empathized, it's time to switch roles. Now it's the Receiver's turn to present whatever is true for them. The Sender becomes the new Receiver—mirroring, validating, and empathizing. The partners will continue to switch roles as needed to make progress on or resolve the issue being discussed.

These steps encourage us to listen deeply to and remain curious about our partner (which, by the way, is part of what Harville and Helen credit for the success and longevity of their own relationship).

They believe the main cause of conflict is objection to difference. We live in our own "inner world," and we think others live and interpret things the same way we do, but that's not the case. And so we become confused as to the how and why of our loved one's state of being, words, and actions.

Helen also said something really interesting during our talk. "People think a relationship is two people with a history," she told me, "but we take pains to say a relationship is two people and the space between." That reminded me of John Grey's "two-brain problem" and the challenges that all relationships face at their core. It's not about one partner or the other, but about the combination, the bringing together of two hearts and minds—with everything that it involves.

Making it work in the "between"—and creating safety for vulnerability there—may just be the secret to happy, emotionally healthy relationships. When working with couples, Helen and Harville focus on four techniques. "One is the dialogue process, where people ask for an appointment to have a dialogue with the other," Dr. Hunt said. "The second is learning to convert a frustration into a request. Number three is having empathy for one another and learning about each other's childhood experiences, wounds, trauma, etc. And number four: daily affirmations. Always try to go to bed giving each other words of appreciation for that day. To create a safe space, the partners must be equals. There should be zero negativity and lots of empathy."

Harville had another item to add to this list: playfulness. He spoke about a Mayo Clinic study of happy, thriving couples. "The indicator, the primary feature, is spontaneous play, not structured play," he said, sharing that when he and Helen were working on their relationship at one point, they did a lot of structured play. But it wasn't doing the trick. "Spontaneous play is when you walk into the room and you start playing—maybe just dancing to a song on the radio—and the person joins. When you're playing like this, your neurochemical system is filled with endorphins and sometimes with dopamine, but you can't get those chemicals to run through your stream if you're scared and feel unsafe, because then you have cortisol and adrenalin. Spontaneous play is the feature of the best relationships and it helps to quickly repair distress."

Speaking of distress, experts say that when we find ourselves in a heated discussion, we can prevent the argument from escalating by agreeing, with our partner, to continue the conversation by lying down on a bed or even the floor. It sends signals of safety and rest to our brains and works as a damper for anger.

What truly matters in a relationship is that you feel like equals. As John Grey put it, "Do you feel you're very important to your partner? Do you feel your feelings matter to your partner? Do you feel valued by your partner?" He even suggested taking it one step further: "Say that's your wedding vow: 'We will emotionally repair everything, and how we know it's repaired [is] because we'll both feel repaired.'"

We can all take this advice and make up new vows—whether we're married or not—and the next time we get into it with our partner, we can try a different approach to conflict resolution and lie down on the floor!

Breaking Out of the (Attachment-Style) Box

WITH DR. JOHN GREY

As we've seen, our strategies for how to emotionally interact with a significant other were wired into our brains before we even had words. We've also learned that, as adults, we may unconsciously act out the insecurities of our attachment styles. It's helpful, then, to become aware of how these styles may be operating within us and between us. As they say, you must see the box before you can get out of the box. Taking personal inventory can help. Speaking of boxes, check the box next to any of the statements below that apply to you.

ATTACHMENT INVENTORY—LIST A

- ☐ Growing up, I did not talk about my feelings much, if at all.
- ☐ I was raised to be self-soothing and self-sufficient.
- ☐ I am not emotionally needy like other people.
- ☐ I like to have a lot of alone time.
- ☐ Sometimes I have difficulty reconnecting after being alone.
- ☐ I'm proud of being the independent type.
- ☐ I can get overwhelmed discussing feelings.
- ☐ I tend to distance or shut down around upset emotions.
- ☐ If only my partner would be happy and stop complaining, I'd be happy.
- ☐ I usually withdraw when I am in distress.
- ☐ I take care of my own feelings without needing to talk them out.
- ☐ When there are upsets, I like to just move on. I tend to let go of the past.

- ☐ I sometimes feel rejected, unappreciated, or not accepted.
- ☐ When my partner gets upset, my brain tells me things like: "I can never get it right." "I feel like a failure." "Nothing I do is ever enough." "It seems hopeless." "I don't want to rock the boat."
- ☐ When there is triggering or upset, I tend to do one or more of these: withdraw, distance, avoid, ignore, shut down, try to rationalize, debate, use logic, dismiss feelings.

ATTACHMENT INVENTORY—LIST B

- ☐ Growing up, I got inconsistent responses when I was upset.
- ☐ I sometimes had to beware of or take care of a parent's emotional states.
- ☐ I am a feeling person and I am very expressive.
- ☐ I yearn to be emotionally close and connected with my partner.
- ☐ Sometimes I have difficulty separating after being together.
- ☐ I am a people person and am good at talking about relationships and feelings.
- ☐ I like to engage in discussions about how I and others feel.
- ☐ I want to fully discuss upsets or issues with my partner.
- ☐ To be happy, I need my partner to open up, be present, and address what we really feel.
- ☐ It makes me more upset if my partner avoids or distances.
- ☐ I need to talk about my feelings when I'm distressed.
- ☐ When there are upsets, I tend to pursue my partner. I want to talk it all out.
- ☐ I tend to focus on whether my partner is really here with me or not.

- ☐ I question whether I am as important to my partner as my partner is to me.
- ☐ I sometimes feel abandoned, disconnected, unimportant, or that my feelings don't matter.
- ☐ When upset, my brain tells me things like: "My feelings don't matter." "I'm all alone." "I am not sure I really matter." "I come last on my partner's priority list." "It's like I'm invisible."
- ☐ When I'm upset, I tend to do one or more of these: pursue, pressure, push, prod, provoke, interrogate, complain, criticize, blow up.

All done? Now compare the number of boxes you checked in each list. List A includes typical features of an island. List B includes features of a wave. You may be clearly one or the other, or a mix of both.

Below are some suggestions to help you expand beyond the limits of your attachment style. To get a different result, you move beyond your wired-in impulses and, in some ways, start doing the opposite of what your usual reaction pattern would dictate. This does not change who you are, but it is a starting place for expanding your emotional repertoire.

IF YOU ACT LIKE AN ISLAND WHEN THERE ARE UPSETS: Instead of avoiding or distancing, turn toward your partner and share in addressing the distress. Place value on interdependence and provide distress relief. Learn to put words to the deeper things going on in you that are emotionally distressing.

IF YOU ACT LIKE A WAVE WHEN THERE ARE UPSETS: Instead of letting feelings escalate, put on the brakes. Rather than pursuing or criticizing, slow down and self-regulate. Speak from your vulnerable core. Reach out more directly and simply for what you need. Realize your partner is also in distress and provide relief.

You can also make rules with your partner about how to better handle upsets and triggering. You might agree to notice if either of you is in distress, and then slow down or pause together. At a minimum, calm down and get back to your best self. Even better, say or do something to calm each other—perhaps "We're okay here. We will repair this." Then, once you are back in your best self, engage in an effective process of emotional repair so you can reconnect and collaborate to resolve the issue at hand in a win-win fashion.

Relationship Advice for the End of the Patriarchy

All this advice is inspiring and practical, but it works only if both partners are all in. In our society, however, where men are too often taught that being vulnerable and open about their feelings makes them somehow "less than masculine," it can be hard to get to a place where both partners are willing to do what it takes to build and repair a healthy, loving relationship.

Terry Real has spent a lot of time thinking about men and the ways they can sometimes struggle with intimacy, connection, and vulnerability, and how this can have such a profound effect on relationships. He has thoughtful ideas about how to achieve intimacy when one partner might not be as far along that path as the other, and an inspiring vision about what relationships might look like in a post-patriarchy world. We started out talking about heterosexual relationships, but his excellent advice isn't limited by gender, sexual identity, or sexual preference.

Sophie Grégoire: Do women—because we have great responsibility, and pressure, in nurturing relationships—need to give and offer intimacy to men, even if they're not ready yet? And let's be clear here: there are many open-hearted men who are seeking this—and all men need it, as all humans need it. But is it our responsibility to give it even if they are not?

Terry Real: Women are socialized to know more about relationships and, for many, to want more from relationships than men are socialized to. So there's an asymmetry. And the Catch-22 for the woman is, "If I don't teach the guy how to step up for me, I don't get it; if I do teach him, I get embroiled in his autonomy issues and he feels like I'm condescending and bossing around, and I still don't get it, but now it's my fault." So, you recognize that?

SG: Oh yes [laughs].

TR: Here is the way out: humility. Resist the temptation of teaching your guy how to be more relational because you're more expert at that than he is. Resist the temptation of being the voice of objective reality and authority.

SG: A lot of women, when we talk about relationships, feel like we have to watch over our men and take care of them. We're nurturers; we're carers—and then we feel undernurtured in return.

TR: There are three phases of getting what you want in a relationship. This is particularly important, I think, for women. The first phase I call "daring to rock the boat." This is the assertive phase; this is where you grab your partner by the collar and you say, "You'd better listen up: this is really important to me. This ain't going away; this is serious."

Once your partner is listening, drop the aggression—everybody gets this wrong. Stop criticizing the poor guy. Drop the sword and shield, roll up your sleeves, and help out. That's relational—no one does that. The relational golden rule is "What could I give you to help you give me what I'm asking for?" And who does that?

And number three is making it worth their while. Once they start to give it to you, reward them; don't criticize them. And

151

everybody gets that wrong, too. I teach people to celebrate the glass 15 percent full.

In relational life therapy, the method I've created, I see it as equal parts therapy and social change. Moving men, women, and nonbinary people into intimacy is synonymous with moving them beyond patriarchy, because patriarchy is not built for intimacy. Intimacy is a new demand, historically. We never wanted an intimate marriage before. Go look at Western literature; all passionate relationships were adulterous.

The idea of a passionate, long-term lover relationship is brand new historically, but we don't teach our kids the skills they need to pull it off. I teach people how to stand up for themselves with love—that's brand new—how to cherish your partner and stand up for yourself at the same time—that's beyond patriarchy. I teach people how to listen to their partners non-defensively and with compassion, and then to repair. People don't know how to do that.

The first thing is understanding the difference between the child part of you that learned to adapt and the wise adult part of you. And then beginning to form a relationship with the adaptive child part of you. I teach my students to always be respectful of the exquisite intelligence of the adaptive child. But I have a saying: adaptive then, maladaptive now. You did just what you needed to do, but you're not that four-year-old girl, your partner is not your father, and you can dare do something different today.

SG: There are probably a lot of people out there who have very good relationships, good intimacy, but you also talk about the difference between good intimacy and fierce intimacy. What does that mean?

TR: I don't think you can have real, good intimacy without being fierce. "Fierce intimacy" means that you take each other on, that you deal, that you don't let things fester.

Under patriarchy, you're either accommodating or you're powerful, but you can't be both at the same time. And moving beyond patriarchy is being connected and being powerful in the same breath. That's brand new. I call it "loving power" or "soft power," and it's beyond patriarchy.

It's the difference between saying, "Sophie, don't talk to me like that"—that is fair enough—and saying, "Sophie, I want to hear what you have to say; could you change your tone and bring it down a little so I can actually listen to it?" Two ways of saying the same thing, but one's about me, me, me, me, me, and the other is about us.

You can be powerful and cherish your relationship at the same time, but we have to learn how. And doing that brings us beyond the culture of individualism and patriarchy—it's a new frontier. "Let me love you and teach you how to do this differently for me"—both in the same breath.

How to Get What You Want out of Your Relationship
WITH TERRY REAL

In his book *The New Rules of Marriage*, Terry Real describes five strategies that definitely *don't* work when it comes to getting what you want out of your relationship, especially during times of conflict. Do any of these sound familiar?

- Insisting on being right (or arguing about whose point of view is more accurate)
- Controlling your partner (directly or indirectly, through manipulation)
- Speaking before you think (with no kindness or respect)
- Retaliating (being passive-aggressive or trying to inflict the same kind of pain we are feeling)
- Withdrawing (an "I'm out and I don't care" attitude)

I'd be lying if I said I'd never fallen into any of these traps (and I expect you would be, too). So how can we do better? Thankfully, Terry also has five "winning" strategies that we can add to our relationship toolbox.

- Shift from complaint to request: learn how to ask mindfully for what you want and need.
- Speak to repair with love and respect: engage in a loving dialogue where both partners feel safe, and then let go of the outcome.
- Listen with compassion: you don't have to agree on everything, but you do have to be curious and understanding.
- Empower each other: give as much as you can, and make sure to acknowledge what your partner gives.
- Cherish each other: give positive feedback, invest time and energy into your relationship, give back to the world together.

If you think back to the beginning of this chapter—where we talked about love and all its amazing benefits—you'll recall that we also acknowledged how difficult relationships can be to sustain. It takes work, sometimes hard work, to get it right. But think about how you feel when you're in deep connection with your partner, or even a friend—when you feel safe in their presence, able to be your authentic self and know that that's enough. Isn't that feeling worth some work? "A couple's history is worth saving," John Grey says. He's right.

He is excited about studies that are working with pairs of brains and looking at how they influence each other. When I asked him what we could learn from that, this is what he said:

JG: I think there has to be a Declaration of Interdependence at some point if we're going to make it as a species. And that's what I'm talking about for a couple. And so, what are the terms of that? We repair everything emotionally. We collaborate until everything's successful, win-win, no matter how hard that is to achieve. We regulate each other when things become upsetting. Imagine if countries did that with each other.

The organic one-on-one is the most powerful thing around. And it always will be. I know that out of my personal experience. I know that out of working with couples in my intensive marriage retreats for the last thirty years. Forty years together, totally out of sorts, relationship's at the end, and they come, hang with me for three days, and they go home in love. There's my data.

SG: I think that message is so reassuring, because it tells us that we'll only get out of it together.

JG: Well, yeah, we're in it together. That's one of the mantras of interdependency. We're in it together. We're in each other's care.

Who among us doesn't like to be cared for? We are biologically wired for it, after all. And yet most of us would agree that partnership and marriage is far from easy. This is why we must feed our relationships by becoming kinder, more curious, and more compassionate with our partner.

While warm relationships are stress regulators, not all of these relationships need to be linked to a romantic partner. In the next chapter, we explore how we can enlarge our circle of healthy relationships and raise our kids to do the same, for the health and well-being of all.

Finding Your Attachment Style

As we've seen throughout this chapter, the bond of attachment we form with our parents or caregivers in our first years is, without a doubt, a key feature in our emotional landscape. I seem to be "securely attached" with some "anxious preoccupied" mixed in. What about you? The quiz below, taken from the bestselling book *Attached: The New Science of Adult Attachment and How It Can Help You Find—and Keep—Love* by Amir Levine and Rachel S. F. Heller, provides an opportunity to explore your own attachment style. Check the small box next to each statement that is true for you. If the answer is untrue, don't mark the item at all.

	TRUE		
	A	B	C
I often worry that my partner will stop loving me.	☐		
I find it easy to be affectionate with my partner.		☐	
I fear that once someone gets to know the real me, s/he won't like who I am.	☐		
I find that I bounce back quickly after a breakup. It's weird how I can just put someone out of my mind.			☐
When I'm not involved in a relationship, I feel somewhat anxious and incomplete.	☐		
I find it difficult to emotionally support my partner when s/he is feeling down.			☐

	TRUE		
	A	B	C
When my partner is away, I'm afraid that s/he might become interested in someone else.	☐		
I feel comfortable depending on romantic partners.		☐	
My independence is more important to me than my relationships.			☐
I prefer not to share my innermost feelings with my partner.			☐
When I show my partner how I feel, I'm afraid s/he will not feel the same about me.	☐		
I am generally satisfied with my romantic relationships.		☐	
I don't feel the need to act out much in my romantic relationships.		☐	
I think about my relationships a lot.	☐		
I find it difficult to depend on romantic partners.			☐
I tend to get very quickly attached to a romantic partner.	☐		
I have little difficulty expressing my needs and wants to my partner.		☐	
I sometimes feel angry or annoyed with my partner without knowing why.			☐

	TRUE		
	A	B	C
I am very sensitive to my partner's moods.	☐		
I believe most people are essentially honest and dependable.		☐	
I prefer casual sex with uncommitted partners to intimate sex with one partner.			☐
I'm comfortable sharing my personal thoughts and feelings with my partner.		☐	
I worry that if my partner leaves me, I might never find someone else.	☐		
It makes me nervous when my partner gets too close.			☐
During a conflict, I tend to impulsively do or say things I later regret, rather than be able to reason about things.	☐		
An argument with my partner doesn't usually cause me to question our entire relationship.		☐	
My partners often want me to be more intimate than I feel comfortable being.			☐
I worry that I'm not attractive enough.	☐		
Sometimes people see me as boring because I create little drama in relationships.		☐	

	TRUE		
	A	B	C
I miss my partner when we're apart, but then when we're together, I feel the need to escape.			☐
When I disagree with someone, I feel comfortable expressing my opinions.		☐	
I hate feeling that other people depend on me.			☐
If I notice that someone I'm interested in is checking out other people, I don't let it faze me. I might feel a pang of jealousy, but it's fleeting.		☐	
If I notice that someone I'm interested in is checking out other people, I feel relieved—it means s/he's not looking to make things exclusive.			☐
If I notice that someone I'm interested in is checking out other people, it makes me feel depressed.	☐		
If someone I've been dating begins to act cold and distant, I may wonder what's happened, but I'll know it's probably not about me.		☐	
If someone I've been dating begins to act cold and distant, I'll probably be indifferent; I might even be relieved.			☐
If someone I've been dating begins to act cold and distant, I'll worry that I've done something wrong.	☐		

	TRUE		
	A	B	C
If my partner was to break up with me, I'd try my best to show her/him what s/he is missing (a little jealousy can't hurt).	☐		
If someone I've been dating for several months told me s/he wants to stop seeing me, I'd feel hurt at first, but I'd get over it.		☐	
Sometimes when I get what I want in a relationship, I'm not sure what I want anymore.			☐
I won't have much of a problem staying in touch with my ex (strictly platonic)—after all, we have a lot in common.		☐	

Add up all your checked boxes in column A: _____

Add up all your checked boxes in column B: _____

Add up all your checked boxes in column C: _____

SCORING KEY

The more statements that you check in a category, the more you will display characteristics of the corresponding attachment style. Category A represents the *anxious* attachment style, category B represents the *secure* attachment style, and category C represents the *avoidant* attachment style.

ANXIOUS: You love to be very close to your romantic partners and have the capacity for great intimacy. You often fear, however, that your partner does not wish to be as close as you would like him or her to be. Relationships tend to consume a large part of your emotional energy. You tend to be very sensitive to small fluctuations in your partner's moods and actions, and although your senses are often accurate, you take your partner's behaviours too personally. You experience a lot of negative emotions within the relationship and get easily upset. As a result, you tend to act out and say things you later regret. If the other person provides a lot of security and reassurance, however, you are able to shed much of your preoccupation and feel contented.

SECURE: Being warm and loving in relationships comes naturally to you. You enjoy being intimate without becoming overly worried about your relationships. You take things in stride when it comes to romance and don't get easily upset over relationship matters. You effectively communicate your needs and feelings to your partner and are strong at reading your partner's emotional cues and responding to them. You share your successes and problems with your mate and are able to be there for him or her in times of need.

AVOIDANT: It is very important for you to maintain your independence and self-sufficiency, and you often prefer autonomy to intimate relationships. Even though you do want to be close to others, you feel uncomfortable with too much closeness and tend to keep your partner at arm's length. You don't spend much time worrying about your romantic relationships or about being rejected. You tend not to open up to your partners, and they often complain that you are emotionally distant. In relationships, you are often on high alert for any signs of control or impingement on your territory by your partner.

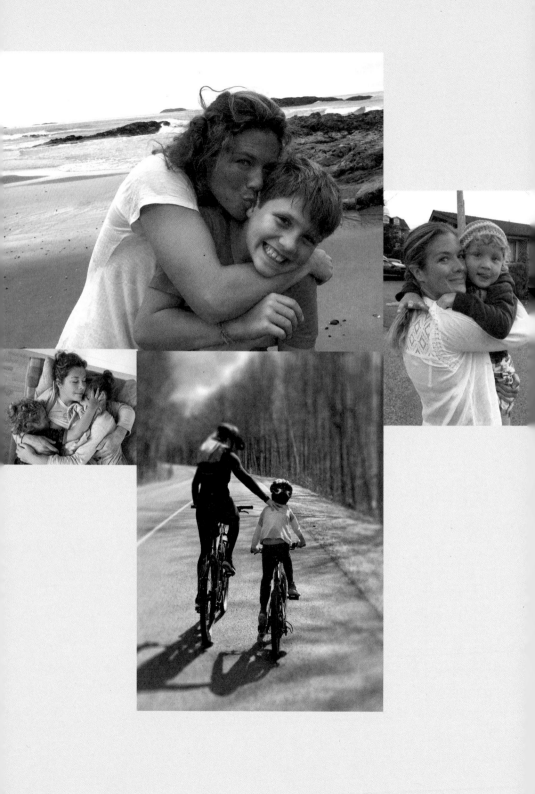

6

Widening the Circle

It Takes a Family

I am a person through other people. My humanity is tied to yours.

ZULU PROVERB—UBUNTU

It's six in the morning as I write this. We're on a family vacation, and I'm sitting at the dining room table with my computer open. I didn't sleep well. We'd had a wonderful day all together, but it ended in an unresolved argument with the kids after dinner. Never go to bed angry! My monkey brain kept jumping from one thought to another, wondering where I might have gone wrong as a mother, or if there were things I should have picked up on sooner with my children, emotionally speaking. Had I been listening enough, or been too quick to judge? Should we look to a therapist for support when we hit rough patches, or just manage things on our own? The list goes on and on.

My mind flashes back to the night before and our discussion at dinner. I can still hear the raised voices, the "I can't take this anymore," the lack of gratitude, the incessant debating, the anger, the tears, the feeling of not being understood and not being free. And I get it, I really do. I remember feeling the same way at their age. As we've seen, teenagers have a deep need to be heard, and their rebellious behaviour is a healthy sign that they are forging their own personality. I'm a pretty open-minded, fun, and in-tune mom, and I encourage my kids to get out there and explore the world. That said, I also have solid principles, and I want my children to grow up with an appreciation of life and a respect for all beings. I long for them to develop self-compassion so they can offer it to others. I wish upon them unconditional love and lasting friendships. Easier said than done, right? Especially as I know that part of this journey to full, authentic, and compassionate adulthood belongs to *them* now, and not to me anymore.

And yet I have been their anchor since their birth, and have been physically present at almost every school drop-off and pick-up. I offer them love and support at every step. I've spent a lot of time alone with them and sacrificed parts of my professional journey to raise them. How do I know, as they move into new stages in their lives, how much to weigh in on and how much to let go? How do I know when to pay more attention to my own well-being, as they learn to take care of their own? How can I be the best mother, friend, partner, and worker I can be? And what happens when I make a mistake and the whole world sees it?

Great, I feel another night of disturbed sleep coming on . . . !

Tending to the Roots

To every parent out there, let me just say this: it sure ain't easy, right? Actually, that message extends to anyone who has a hand in raising, teaching, mentoring, or otherwise nurturing the kids in our lives. It's a big job—a hugely important job—and there are days when we feel up to it and days when we're not sure we're doing anything right.

When I'm having moments of doubt, I try to remember that we're all human. It's so easy to forget that, as we work like machines, following the incessant rhythm of *métro-boulot-dodo*, as we say in French ("the rat race" in English). Most of us are trying so hard to do it all that we forget a crucial fact: when it comes to loving and nourishing relationships, we can only move forward from the starting place of our own emotional journey. As we've learned, we must understand our hard-wiring in order to understand how we function in all our relationships. And make no mistake: parenting *is* a relationship. As Gordon Neufeld explains, "The biggest mistake we've made is to focus on parenting—which is actually a fairly new construct—as something you do, rather than as someone you are to the child. Context is everything. It is so important even in adolescence for our children to be attached to us. Because just like a plant, that's the roots. The flourishing is what we see. It's the roots that we don't see where the story lies."

That's huge, right? If we think of parenting as a relationship, it means that when we interact with our children, our brains and nervous systems are constantly being triggered and nourished (or undernourished) by the other. And that other has the power to place us right in front of our most profound truths, which can reveal flaws and pain. We often say that kids know how to "push our buttons," but that's not quite right. It's more like they challenge us to be better and more patient, to be compassionate, playful, attentive, and perseverant.

Kids want the attention and true presence of the adults in their lives. But we all get so busy with our jobs, lives, and problems that we sometimes forget that the real work we must do is to slow down and check in with our own emotions on a daily basis. I have lost my patience more than once with my kids, but I rarely get mad at them or easily irritated after I've meditated, for example. When I slow down, I'm more in tune with my own emotions and struggles. I am suddenly better positioned to listen, and I feel as if I have a deep well of patience. This helps me remember how important the depth and consistency of our presence actually is.

Thinking about this now, it strikes me that I didn't need reminding to go slow when I was pregnant, or in the days after my children were born. I just knew how precious that time was. We'd been struggling to conceive for about two years, since 2005. I was working for CTV (and continued to until 2010), and so much was going on in our lives. I vividly recall sitting on the couch one night, watching TV, with tears rolling down my face. Justin turned to me and said, "No, Sophie, your ovaries are not 'shrivelled-up little raisins'!" He was repeating a line from the show we'd been watching, because he knew exactly what I thought when I heard it. Finally, we attended a fertility clinic and both of us went through a series of tests. When everything came back "all clear," the doctor told us to stop "trying," or even thinking about trying, and just let nature take its course. (I must have thrown out at least a dozen negative pregnancy tests by then).

Meanwhile, my brother-in-law, Sacha, and his partner, Zoe, announced that they were expecting. We were over the moon. I sometimes wonder if the happiness I felt for them and the pure joy that flooded my heart the moment I held that beautiful baby in my arms caused a switch to flip in my brain and my body. A month later, something felt different, and I just knew.

Over the next nine months, I gained about twenty-five pounds and felt more beautiful, alive, magical, sensuous, and empowered than I'd ever felt. Don't worry, I'm not going to tell you it was perfect. Pregnancy came with plenty of challenges, from intense nausea and regular Braxton Hicks contractions to varicose veins, hemorrhoids, and more. But I was determined to stay healthy and active. One of my regular walking routes took me up the hundreds of stairs on Mont-Royal. I'd begin by crossing the cemetery, which reminded me of the uncertainty and preciousness of life. But sometimes basic needs got in the way of deep thoughts. I was always hungry in those days. (My worst craving? Steamed hot dogs. So bad. I can't tell you how much I wished it was something healthier, but what can I say? Those steamies were *just* salty enough.) One day, while out walking with my mom, I was so famished that I actually asked the grounds-keepers if they had anything I could possibly snack on. One of them pulled his lunch box out of their truck and gave me his homemade sandwich. I didn't want to deprive him of his lunch, but he wouldn't take no for an answer. I could have kissed him. Thankfully, my mom held me back!

Oh, the joys of carrying another human in your belly. It is one of the most intimate and life-affirming experiences I've ever had. Maybe that's why I had three children. You forget the difficult parts. It's like everything made sense to me during that time. I suddenly felt connected to other women and mothers in a way I'd never known I could feel. And I was so in tune with my own body as well. We hadn't asked to know the sex of the baby—we wanted to be surprised—but I was convinced I was having a boy. I was right. In October 2007, after eighteen hours of labour, Xavier was born. It felt as if the whole world was spinning inside that room. Nothing else mattered. I'd been in love with him ever since I'd found out I was pregnant, but that love grew exponentially the moment I saw him. I just wanted to hold him close to me forever. I was also a little bit scared. I knew without a doubt that I wanted to be a mom; like most new parents, though, I wasn't sure if I had all it would take to be a *good* mom. But there was no turning back, and we soon settled into a routine as a family.

The days after my children were born were some of the happiest of my life. I felt at one with every living thing, and especially connected to my babies as we gazed at each other during breastfeeding and quiet time spent cuddling. Like most moms, I was also exhausted, and breastfeeding came with some hiccups, but my mind felt quiet and full at the same time. I was satiated in every way. The inner peace I experienced then reminded me of how blissful and untethered I could feel while practising yoga and meditation, which I had started before getting pregnant with Xavier. I was so aware that I was beginning a new journey—one that would change both me and the family

Justin and I were building. I couldn't wait to see where it would take me, and I had no idea how much I would learn along the way.

Psychologist Rose-Marie Charest has a wealth of knowledge when it comes to understanding and guiding family dynamics. She's seen hundreds of individuals and family members scrambling to make sense of difficult relationships, like so many of us do, and she believes that mental health is a responsibility shared by family, school, society, organizations, and individuals. I couldn't agree more. We had such an interesting conversation about parenting, and families, and mentors, and . . . Just listen in!

> **Sophie Grégoire:** In thinking about the attachment relationship and how important it is for brain and nervous system development, I'm wondering if it's a bit like we are teaching our children to develop parental tenderness toward themselves.
>
> **Rose-Marie Charest:** Absolutely. That's what we need to learn. Gradually, we become our own parent, hopefully a good one. We will still need outside support, but we integrate this ability to trust ourselves. We must also learn how to relax and realize how much our thinking can influence our emotions, our interpersonal relationships, and our entire affective life. To be able to trust others, one must have self-compassion; otherwise, expectations toward others will be too high. I've had a clinical practice for forty years, and the most unhappy people I have seen are those who can't trust anyone. When you can't trust anyone, you are bound for loneliness.
>
> **SG:** One of your mentors told you, "Listen, there are basically two categories of people in the world: those who are suffering because they didn't have a family and those who are suffering because of their family." Is objecting to difference, the fact that we don't all think alike, one of the greatest sources of conflict in families?

RC: Yes. And the more fragile we are, the more intolerant we are of difference. It's true in families and it's true in society. If I want to reduce intolerance, I need to treat the other with kindness. A healthy family is one that accepts individuation, which is the process we go through to become adults. We gradually detach from family by becoming increasingly an individual, and this goes smoothly when attachment to the family is not threatened. Secure attachment is even reinforced, but the person is not required to stay stuck in the family to maintain the attachment; they can move away from it.

SG: How important is it for our young people to have role models who understand themselves and can understand others?

RC: I gave a conference not long ago to an entire education network, people in school settings, and I told them how much having a role model is a factor that fosters their psychological health. Another factor is having opportunities for success. We need to stop putting children in moulds. And we need to try to limit how much we do that with adults, too, and instead look at what each person can succeed at. Because self-esteem isn't supported just by compliments from others. It has to be supported by experience, and a person who experiences success has self-confidence.

SG: Everyone has little spats or arguments in their family. Up to what point is that normal? Are more dramatic breaks ever warranted?

RC: People I've seen break definitively with their families are rarely very happy with having done that. I tend to think that in some cases when the family is truly toxic, when there is a real impediment, it's better to put some distance in the relationship rather than ending it. People who break ties with their parents think about it often, but in some cases, they don't have a choice. That was the avenue they needed to take because it was just too destructive. But in most cases, it's better to get perspective about what is going on in the family rather than dramatizing with a split. Rupture is experienced as a trauma not just for the person who is rejected but also for the person who does the rejecting as well.

We have to ask: What is a relationship? A relationship is three parts: it's my territory, the other's territory, and our shared territory. I don't need to share all these territories with all members of my family. I'm from a family of eight kids. I often go on vacation with one of my sisters; with another one we share books and with another one we discuss the arts. I wouldn't try to do every activity with every member of my family.

SG: That's a big gang! [Laughs.]

RC: It's too big a gang to do everything together! [Laughs.]

SG: We know how important communication is in relationships. How can families communicate better to avoid those dramatic ruptures?

RC: I think the best communication exercise I can recommend for a family is to find a project that everyone wants to work on. It can be a tiny project, but it has to be unifying and take us outside ourselves to make others feel good, too.

SG: That could be anything from planning a veggie garden to volunteering together once a month with elders in need to repurposing a room in your home into a family game space for more time together to starting a family book club, right?

RC: Yes. There are so many options. We know that happy people are people with projects, and even more so when these are collective projects. Another exercise when there is unease in a family is to start by asking, "How can I approach the other with compassion?" The approach needs to be made without criticism and/or the accumulated frustration that could lead to an explosion.

Speaking with Rose-Marie made me realize that the more aware we are of our emotions, the better equipped we will be when the time comes to mend small ruptures in our families. Imagine if we could approach these "explosions in progress" with calm and rational heads and tame them before anyone gets hurt? That would definitely help me in my life. There's obviously a learning curve to surmount here, and some trial and error along the way, but that's life, isn't it? It's okay to feel our way through, as long as we remain vulnerable, honest, and open to learning. I can be stubborn at times, but I've realized that it gets me nowhere, so I'm much more mindful of it as I age.

Putting the Pieces Together

Speaking of learning, let's connect some of the puzzle pieces we've been collecting over the last few chapters. We've seen how critical our childhood bonds of attachment are in terms of shaping our emotional landscape and our ability to thrive (or not) in relationships throughout our lives. We also know that parenting is not a role, as we so often think, but a relationship. Put those two pieces together and the picture starts to take shape: we bring more than a little bit of our own childhood into our relationship with our children. The ways in which we choose to parent are intrinsically tied up with how we ourselves were parented. But that's not to say we're locked in. We can learn and grow and parent more mindfully than perhaps our parents did with us.

Dr. Shefali Tsabary, who goes by Dr. Shefali, is an expert in family dynamics and personal development, teaches courses around the globe, and has written five books, three of which have been *New York Times* bestsellers. Her two landmark titles—*The Conscious Parent* and *The Awakened Family*—have inspired a generation of parents to look harder at their own emotional patterns and embrace a different way of parenting. I asked her how our bonds of attachment influence our parenting style.

Dr. Shefali Tsabary: Our childhood attachment patterns, traumas, and conditioning are the three primary influencers of our parenting belief systems and attitudes toward our kids. Unless we heal these past patterns through inner work and growth, we will unavoidably dump our "emotional crap" onto our kids without conscious awareness, thereby repeating generational patterns of pain and trauma.

Sophie Grégoire: What's the first step toward doing better? How can we become calmer and more aware parents?

ST: There are many deep-rooted ideologies that have conditioned parents the world over to adopt habituated belief systems that are quite toxic and dysfunctional for the well-being of our children. The first step is to let go of the belief system that we need to control our children's creation into perfect, happy beings. When the resulting unrealistic expectations don't materialize, we get angry at our children. We feel like failures, and so do they. Once we're aware of how this belief around control is contaminating our relationship with our children, we can begin to let it go and work on building strong connections with them. It all starts when we awaken to our own inner lack and insecurities that require us to have control in the first place. [For more about these habituated notions, see "Debunking the Myths of Parenting" on page 174.]

SG: What's the biggest lesson you've learned from kids? From parents?

ST: The biggest lesson our children teach us is to live in the present moment in an authentic and unconditioned manner. No human knows how to do this better than young children. This is why I call them our greatest awakeners and teachers. Sadly, we don't think they are, and therefore fail to learn from these master gurus.

The biggest lesson I have learned from parents, unfortunately, is about the unmitigated and unrelenting nature of the human ego. And how if we don't heal our childhood patterns, we will pass on generational trauma to our kids without our aware-ness, cycling them through the same pain we went through and not realizing one bit of it until our children or we fall apart.

SG: What do you tell parents who come to you and ask, "How do we get our kids to listen to us?" Should the question really be "Can we listen to them better?"

ST: It is not our children's job to listen to us. It's not about what they do at all, really. It is *our* job to connect to them in a manner where they partner with us effortlessly. In this partnership, mutual listening happens as a by-product, not a prerequisite. When parents shift from wanting to control their kids—"Listen to me; follow me; do as I say; etc."—to "How can I listen and attune to you well enough that you and I synergize effort-lessly?" then the entire dynamic shifts from a hierarchical, top-down model to a mutual, reciprocal relationship.

SG: That sounds perfect, but what happens when we mess up? Because we all mess up now and again. Can we repair broken relationships with our kids?

ST: Of course we can. But it's not about mere words of apology. It's about transforming life patterns at the deeper level of inner healing and transformation. Children break relationships because they have felt disavowed and degraded. When we feel seen and understood within a relationship, we will never leave.

SG: How can we help our children foster a better sense of worth?

ST: We can do this when we remove the tentacles of our parental control and expectations and allow our children to be seen, honoured, and celebrated for who it is they are in their essence, removed from what they do, produce, or achieve. When a child feels honoured for who it is they are, then they develop a deep sense of worth.

Debunking the Myths of Parenting

WITH DR. SHEFALI

As we parent or mentor the young people in our lives, we find ourselves up against deeply ingrained ideas that can be hard to shake. In *The Awakened Family*, Dr. Shefali explores how we can move past these outdated notions and into an era of conscious parenting where we feel empowered to make mindful, emotionally aware decisions about raising our children. It all starts with debunking some popular parenting myths.

PARENTING IS ABOUT THE CHILD: This ideology creates behaviours within the parents that cause them to be hyper-focused on raising the perfect child and producing the ideal childhood. This creates a dangerous manic obsession with all aspects of the child's behaviours. This micromanagement stifles the child's innate ability to discover their own path in an autonomous and empowered way. Conscious parenting debunks this myth and turns the spotlight away from the child and onto the parent. Here, parenting is about raising the parent equally and before raising the child. The parents examine themselves and how they project their needs and expectations onto the child. This transfer of focus releases the child to a path of liberation and autonomy.

PARENTING IS ABOUT RAISING A HAPPY AND SUCCESSFUL CHILD: There is no greater disservice we can unleash on our children than this idea that they should be happy and successful. Why? Both of these qualities are highly subjective and almost unrealistic to achieve unless one wears a false persona that's created to please another versus the self. Conscious parenting debunks these goals of the traditional parenting model by focusing on the child's authentic experience of their reality.

PARENTING IS ABOUT CONTROL: The traditional parenting model is all about raising kids under the authority of fear, shame, blame, and control. These are the primary tactics used by the traditional parent to coerce and manipulate children to follow their ways and meet their expectations. Conscious parenting challenges parents to replace this unrelenting desire for power over their children with a quest for connection to their child's essence.

THERE ARE GOOD AND BAD CHILDREN: The traditional parenting model has long espoused this notion of "good" and "bad," where children are constantly categorized and compartmentalized. Conscious parenting exposes parents to how their unconscious judgments of their children have little to do with the child's actual behaviours and all to do with how these behaviours make their parents feel and their own ego's desire for supremacy, comfort, and control.

THE PARENT IS ENTIRELY SELFLESS AND LOVING: While there certainly are elements of selflessness and love in our parenting, most traditional parenting is about the parents' ego. Conscious parenting is the first model to expose the parent to their ego and debunk this notion that parents have children because they are selfless martyrs. It's a difficult idea for many parents to embrace, because it cuts through their unconsciousness with the sharpest knife of a truth they can't bear to encounter within themselves.

We Can All Parent

As parents simply trying to do our best, we don't always realize that our own motivations may be lurking behind what we ask of our children. In a way, the more selfless we are, the more authentically loving we become. I was moved by Dr. Shefali's words about how we can foster a sense of worth in our children by honouring their essence. We all need this, don't we? Isn't that sense of being seen and appreciated for exactly who we are the very basis of emotional health and well-being?

Thinking about this reminded me of a moment I shared with Ella-Grace when she was about five years old. We were reading a Fancy Nancy book, and, as always, there was a new word to learn. This time, it was *humble*. How do you explain *humble* to a five-year-old? I held her close and gave it my best shot: "Well . . . let's say someone loves to read and they are very good at it. They are also quite nice and generous with their friends, and they are very good at sports and drawing, too. But do they go around telling everybody that? No. They are peaceful and quiet with who they are. They don't need the world to know or to tell them how good and beautiful and talented they are. Do you understand, my love?"

"Of course I do," Ella answered. "That's just like me!"

What was I supposed to say to that? In retrospect, I've realized that what I initially saw as an adorable but fairly mundane parenting moment was anything but. When each of us was a child that age, we learned our value through the eyes of the world. Parents and friends and the wider circle of people in a child's life can either help deepen that natural sovereignty, dilute it, or, in the worst cases, abuse it. Part of our responsibility as parents is to ensure that our kids have trustworthy allies who can walk with them as they figure out who they are and how they fit in the world. This can be a challenge in our current cultural climate, where family units are getting smaller, and where we don't build or take part in communities in the same way previous generations did.

A number of the experts I spoke to while writing this book shared their thoughts on what we stand to lose when our circles are too small. In chapter 2, for example, Gordon Neufeld told the story of the interactions he saw between the elderly and teenagers around a village fountain in Provence, and also described the valuable healing he's witnessed in his work with incarcerated youth and Indigenous elders. Dr. Shefali had thoughts on this issue as well. During our conversation about conscious parenting, I asked her whether our family units are too small, and whether we should enlarge them to include a wider community. Her answer? "The nuclear family is the plague of modern existence and the ruin of our children's well-being. Children should not be raised in the unnatural ways we are raising them—disconnected from the 'tribe' and from nature. In these two fundamental ways—living in nuclear pods and removed from nature, stuck in technological artificialities—we have destroyed our children's attempts at having a childhood. Children today don't have a childhood. This has devastating impacts on their inner well-being and prosperity."

Recently, I had a chance to catch up with my friend Jewel Kilcher (whom you likely know simply as Jewel, the Grammy-nominated singer, songwriter, poet, and philanthropist, and from whom we'll hear more in chapter 8). Two decades ago, she created the Inspiring Children Foundation, a non-profit organization dedicated to helping youth development in underserved communities. The foundation works with kids who come from highly traumatic backgrounds and who are coping with suicidal ideation, extreme anxiety, and depression. When I asked her why so many kids are struggling today, she touched on this same topic:

> **Jewel Kilcher:** We no longer live in a village environment. For the first time in humanity's history, we live in completely separate and isolated ways. And so I think it makes a lot of sense that we feel somewhat fractured or dissociative. We've literally and physically pulled ourselves apart.
>
> I think that as colonization swept across the world, we built an altar to the intellect. You know where they say don't throw out the baby with the bathwater? As we dismantled Indigenous cultures and dismantled our own village cultures and began to prize the intellect, the human heart, the human emotional experience, wasn't considered important.
>
> And so we're now the most technologically advanced society in the history of the species, and yet we're killing ourselves at

unprecedented rates. We advanced in ways we thought were valuable, but we didn't see we were paying an incredible price. We've broken the individual into many, many pieces. And I think most of what we're seeing now in the wellness spaces is, how do we integrate all of these aspects of ourselves?

Food for thought, isn't it? Through my travels, I've had the privilege of witnessing many beautiful mentoring relationships between our youth and older members of our society. But in this modern world—which too often equates "old" with "unwanted" or "ugly"—that bond is at risk. And we are all poorer for it. The togetherness that comes from being part of a community, a togetherness we feel physically and emotionally, is both a gift and a core part of who we are. When I asked Gordon Neufeld about the greatest legacy a parent can give to a child, he told me, "Care and a soft heart." And then he continued: "Being able to feel. Feelings will take care of us, and feelings help us to take care of others. It is where our humanity is. It is where our humanness is. It doesn't guarantee there will be success. It is the bottom line. It is in our nature to seek togetherness. Togetherness and care belong together."

Fostering Positive Relationships with Young People

Whether you're a parent, a teacher, a coach, or a mentor, fostering a positive relationship with the kids in your life is always a top priority. When kids feel happy and secure in their relationships, and appreciated for who they are, they are more likely to know the difference between right and wrong, and to find motivation for good behaviour. So how can we encourage positive relationships? In an article on positive parenting strategies, Prodigy Education offers these five tips to get you on your way:

1. Make expectations clear.
2. Be consistent and reliable.
3. Show affection and appreciation.
4. Seek to understand your child.
5. Encourage curiosity, independence, and personal development.

Part 3

Balance

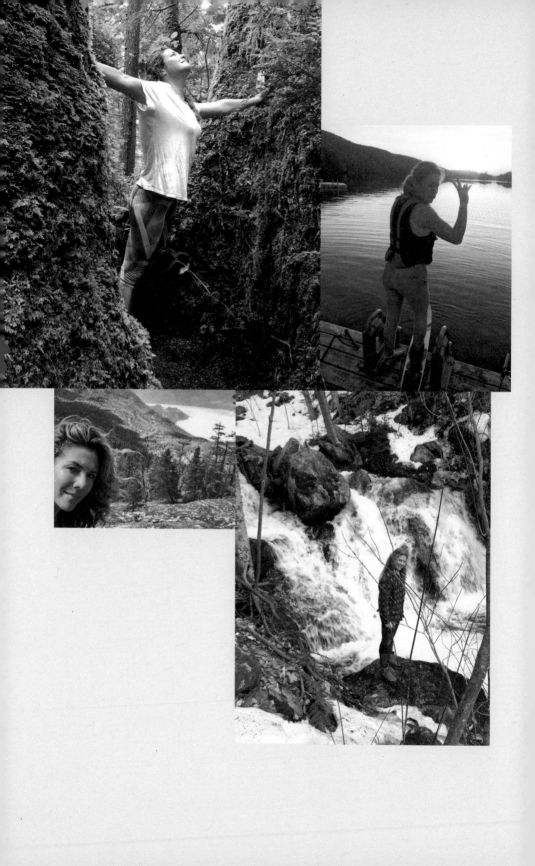

7

Building Blocks for a Strong Foundation

Movement, Nutrition, and Sleep

People say that what we're all seeking is a meaning for life.
I don't think that's what we're really seeking. I think that what
we're seeking is an experience of being alive, so that our life experiences
on the purely physical plane will have resonance with our own innermost
being and reality, so that we actually feel the rapture of being alive.

JOSEPH CAMPBELL

It's a late-fall morning, 2013, and the weather in Montreal is warm and sunny. We've just finished breakfast and I've taken Ella-Grace and Xavier outside to draw with chalk on our driveway and ride their tiny bicycles, outfitted with training wheels. As a mother, it's bizarre to recollect moments like this, in which Hadrien (our "Didi") wasn't yet part of the picture (he was born in 2014). But not having a baby to hold in my arms means I have a bit of freedom to play myself. I hop on my skateboard to practise some very basic tricks—except I am paying more attention to the kids than I am to my own moves! One miscalculation and down I go. My left wrist takes the brunt of the fall, and my

> *Methinks that the moment my legs begin to move, my thoughts begin to flow.*
>
> HENRY DAVID THOREAU

radius breaks in two places. My hand looks like something out of a horror movie. I'm wearing gloves, but there's no way I can get my hand out without fainting from the pain. Justin rushes the kids into the car and off we go to the hospital. They force the bone back into place while I'm dazed on painkillers, and then orthopedics inserts three metal pins and puts me in a cast.

Here's what I knew in those moments: Recovery was going to take a couple of months, and there would have to be some big adjustments. I wouldn't be able to be the (literally) hands-on mom I usually was for the kids. I wouldn't be heading out on the big adventure trek I'd been planning for more than a year. And sure I wouldn't be picking up the guitar anytime soon either! I knew I could adapt to the pain and discomfort, and that I would find ways to parent and cook with one hand, but what affected me most was the fact that I wasn't going to be able to be as physically active. No biking, swimming, skating, skiing. No pulling the kids on their sleds or going sledding myself, for that matter. I knew how much my body would miss moving as much as it normally did, and I also knew the effect that would have on my mood.

I am at my best—physically, mentally, emotionally—when I am active. I don't like to be sedentary. I've always known this about myself, but that period after I broke my wrist really drove it home. And I was reminded of it again while working on this book. Sometimes I felt as if my body and my brain were on totally different tracks. My brain was telling me to stay put and work, but my body was seeking the "experience of being alive" that Joseph Campbell referred to in the quotation at the beginning of this chapter.

Too often, we imagine our mind and our body as separate entities, but they are intrinsically connected. And the way we care for both affects every aspect of our lives, including our capacity for self-love, self-respect, and self-fulfillment. We need physical activity to create a body strong enough to support us in the life we want to lead. We need to nourish that body to keep it healthy. And we need enough rest to allow ourselves time to recharge.

To me, the most important aspect of physical activity is commitment and pleasure. Without finding pleasure in a particular activity, it will be very hard to keep at it. If we all knew a tad more about the mental health benefits of exercise, we might take it more seriously. In working on this chapter, I learned so much about the fascinating science behind movement, nutrition, and sleep. Together, we'll discover what we all have to gain by paying attention to these building blocks that allow us to thrive, and bring more joy into our lives.

Be Moved

When we move physically, we can prepare to be moved emotionally and intellectually. I'm very lucky to have been brought up by a father who taught me how to push my physical boundaries and to enjoy being active in nature and a mother who walked every day to keep fit. Unfortunately, she had a fall in 2023 while out on a beautiful winter walk and broke her kneecap. She moved in with us during her recovery and rehabilitation, and I saw first-hand how less fresh air and movement can affect one's well-being.

The lessons my body and mind learn through moving are precious to me. Take balance, for example. Balance is always key when it comes to moving. A strong body without any flexibility can break, but I now also know that a flexible body without core and overall strength can be injury-prone. Whatever body you have, why not thank it for holding you up, for allowing you to move, to love, to see and taste the world through your senses. Sometimes when I walk down the street, or especially when I'm biking or hiking, I become overwhelmingly aware of how grateful I am for my body. I took it for granted so many times and disconnected from it to my own detriment—especially when I was struggling with eating disorders—but it is still here for me. It has allowed me to carry three babies and hold them close while moving through life, love, adversity, mountains, rivers, and more. My body and I are in a relationship that I nourish and keep showing up for. I guess that's why my body shows up for me, too.

As a former Parks Canada ambassador for newcomers and families, and a FitSpirit ambassador encouraging young Canadian women to become active, I learned that one out of two girls will drop sports during puberty. This is such a shame. The decision to step away from sports and the physical activity that comes with them can have a huge impact on psychological and physical well-being. Although we are a very active family, I still felt a deep reassurance when Ella-Grace enrolled in a dance program in high school, knowing she would be moving her body every day. A week into the program, she told me that the teacher had shown them how to breathe properly. What a gift. We teach people in emergency situations how to breathe to calm their nervous system, and we show women giving birth how to breathe to help control the pain. Why aren't we all making sure that our incredible kids learn more about how they can affect their state of physical and mental well-being by breathing properly? The techniques are easy to learn and could be used prior to an exam, or during times of heartbreak, grief, loss, despair, anger, sadness, and joy, too.

Cyclic Sighing

The next time you feel anxious or stressed, try cyclic sighing. It's my favourite breath technique, and you can do it in just five minutes, if that's all you have. It's also medically proven to enhance mood and calm the nervous system (see the Selected Notes for this chapter, page 291, for more on the study). You can choose to stand up, sit in a chair that supports your back with both feet on the floor, or lie down with support behind your neck. Close your eyes. Relax your mouth, jaw, and forehead. Let go by inhaling deeply through the nose and exhaling fully through the mouth, and then begin:

1. Inhale through the nose for a count of five seconds.
2. Take a tiny extra inhale.
3. Hold your breath for three to five seconds.
4. Exhale through your mouth for eight seconds or longer.

Repeat steps 1 through 4 for five minutes or more at any time of day or night.

Exercising in nature also has tremendous benefits and makes us more aware of our surrounding environment. Research shows that exercising outdoors can boost vitamin D levels, help calm the nervous system, reduce anxiety, and improve mental clarity. Of course, it also burns calories and strengthens muscles. Because we are feeling, social animals, moving freely in the company of other people—in nature or anywhere else—is a bonus. Pairing up with a friend for a bit of activity can be just the motivation you need. I've had some soul-shifting conversations while moving outdoors with friends. Oh, the things we've discussed . . .

When it comes to explaining just how much we can gain from moving our body, Dr. Jennifer J. Heisz has us covered. Jennifer is the author of *Move the Body, Heal the Mind.* She is an associate professor and Canada Research Chair in the Department of Kinesiology at McMaster University, where she directs the NeuroFit Lab. Her award-winning research examines the effects of physical activity on brain function to promote mental health and cognition in young adults, older adults, and individuals with Alzheimer's disease. During our conversation, I learned that she speaks on these issues not only from a place of professional interest but from personal experience. When I asked her how she came to this field of study, this is what she told me:

Dr. Jennifer Heisz: In grad school, I had severe anxiety, some intrusive thoughts, and I went to the doctor and was prescribed an antidepressant, which I was very reluctant to take. Movement didn't come very easily for me, but a friend recommended that I try cycling, and much to my amazement, those bike rides really soothed my mind. It had such a profound effect on me, not just personally—I made exercise a priority—but also professionally. Instead of studying the fundamentals of neuroscience, I shifted the focus of my research to study the amazing impact that exercise has on the brain.

Sophie Grégoire: Why does exercise make us feel better?

JH: Exercise supplies the brain with the vital nutrients it needs to thrive. And when we sit for long periods of time at our desk or in a meeting room or on the couch, the brain gets starved of these vital nutrients. We need to move the muscles, move the body, to get the blood oxygenated and flowing. It releases a ton of neurochemicals in the brain that promote growth, that promote this sense of calm, that help us to manage the stress of everyday life. Exercise releases dopamine—it activates the reward system. Exercising at a somewhat vigorous intensity can also increase endorphins, which are the body's natural painkiller. This is advantageous because it allows us to move through some challenging exercises with minimal pain.

SG: What would you say to people who are thinking, "What, running? I can't even fast-walk, and I'm in chronic pain."

JH: When it comes to movement for mental health, for physical health, every step counts. The benefits can really be felt with minimal movement. So, for someone who's sitting all the time, I recommend taking a two-minute movement break every thirty minutes. Just stand up, stretch, move your body. This helps to increase or counteract the decline in brain blood flow that happens when we sit for long periods of time. Research shows that just a ten-minute self-paced walk can boost creativity, it can boost focus, it can help reduce anxiety, reduce stress, reduce depression.

SG: Actually, let's talk about depression.

JH: One in three people who have depressive symptoms don't actually respond to antidepressant drugs. What the research is showing is that for these individuals in particular, exercise is the medicine they need, and it can have clinically meaningful reductions in their depressive symptoms. And for those who are responding to antidepressant drugs, it's not an either/or situation. Exercise is a really great add-on therapy that can reduce some of the side effects. It can also reduce the dosage that you might have to take of the medication and have really positive overall effects.

SG: What's the relationship between exercise and anxiety?

JH: Exercise has a powerful effect on our feelings of anxiety in the moment. So immediately after we exercise, we have a reprieve from anxiety in this acute phase. Research from my lab shows that thirty minutes of light- to moderate-intensity exercise three times a week is enough to reduce anxiety in people who are feeling anxious.

SG: Some level of inflammation in the body is normal—it's part of our immune system's natural response to infections or wounds—but it can also become harmful if the response lasts for too long. When does exercise help with a necessary anti-inflammatory reaction in the body?

JH: Acute exercise is a little bit inflammatory, and the harder and more intensively you exercise, it can be more inflamma-tory. But immediately after you stop exercising, the muscles release myokines into the blood, which essentially act like an anti-inflammatory cleanup crew. So they clean up all the inflammation that was produced by exercise and then some.

189

So, ultimately, as you continue to exercise your body, it becomes less inflamed. This is important for many different reasons, especially mental health. The anti-inflammatory effects of exercise can help minimize the negative impact that everyday stressors can have on our mental health.

SG: Does exercise allow us to be more resilient from a physiological and psychological perspective?

JH: Psychological stress tends to be imposed on us, uncontrollable, unpredictable, whereas the physical stress of exercise is very much controllable, predictable, and self-selected.

When we think of stress, we always think it's bad, but it's actually very helpful. When we're in a state of stress, the body activates, the brain activates and prepares for battle, but there is also this adaptation and growth that happens. So the body and the brain adapt to this new challenge and they're better able to deal with it when they experience it again. Because there's only one stress response for all stressors, when we challenge the stress response with exercise, it grows stronger for all stressors in our life, including everyday psychological stress. It's this stress resilience, this stress toning, that seems to be really beneficial for helping us navigate our life more calmly, so that when we experience these challenges, we are able to see them as opportunities rather than obstacles. And I think those moments allow people to thrive and reach their full potential.

SG: Can exercise help with healing from post-traumatic stress disorder?

JH: Yes. Partly what happens when we experience trauma is that the body is in a chronic state of stress. So we need to be careful here, because, as we've seen, there's only one stress response for all stressors. If we have a lot of psychological stress in our life, we are not able to tolerate as much physical stress, so you may not necessarily be able to do a vigorous, intensive workout; it may just need to be a walk. But the beautiful thing about exercise is in that period immediately following the workout, you have this reprieve, the stress system comes down and you have this sense of calm, not just for the exercise stress, but all stress in your life. And I see this as a window of opportunity for us to remember what it's like to feel well and to be well, and it gives people a hope that they can then hold on to and bring into the next moment.

SG: What is the relationship between exercise and aging?

JH: As we get older, we do lose some of our cognitive abilities—the brain doesn't regenerate as fast as it used to—but it still has a lot of potential. Our research shows that even if you have a genetic risk for dementia, it doesn't guarantee your fate. Lifestyle matters more than most people think. Physical inactivity can contribute to your dementia risk as much as your genetics. Walking is really beneficial, but if you're a regular walker, you'll probably need to pick up the pace. So you might add some intervals into your walk—increasing the pace between light posts, or adding some hills or even a slow jog, if your fitness can handle that. We know that intermittent walking, preferably on a slight uphill, can get the heart rate up, then we bring it back down with the flat incline, and then we repeat that, and it can significantly improve memory more than regular walking or stretching.

When we exercise in that more intense zone, above the anaerobic threshold, lactate starts to accumulate in the muscles. Typically, we've heard of lactate as a villain—it's often wrongly associated with acidity in the muscles and burning sensations—but lactate might be the hero here. As lactate builds up, it gets into the blood, and it moves to the brain, where it reports to the hippocampus and stimulates the growth of brand-new brain cells by activating a neurochemical. This essentially acts like a fertilizer to support the growth, functioning, and survival of these brand-new brain cells. And so that's an important point: our brain produces brand-new brain cells across the lifespan, even into old age, and we can produce more of those brain cells with exercise.

SG: Let's talk about the relationship between exercise and creativity.

JH: Remember that when you're sitting for prolonged periods of time, the blood flow decreases to the brain. And so the brain is not functioning optimally, and creativity requires a dynamic flexibility within the brain. This is governed partly by the prefrontal cortex, which has two modes. It has focused mode, where it's able to focus your attention on the task and ignore distractions. But it also has this mental flexibility mode, where it can draw from past experiences, combine information, and think divergently, and that requires mental flexibility. We need the combination of the two to be creative and productive at the same time.

Exercising helps to infuse that prefrontal cortex with the nutrients it needs to thrive and perform this suite of executive functions with precision.

SG: What tricks can we use to motivate ourselves to move?

JH: Wake up, put your workout clothes on, and start listening to music you love!

SG: How about a big dance party outdoors as we start the day! [Laughs.]

JH: Yeah! Music stimulates the reward system, gets dopamine primed for the activity. You can also try swishing a sugary drink in your mouth before you exercise—just swish it in your mouth and spit it out, if you want. Research shows it reduces your feelings of exertion, especially during the first part of your workout. And try exercising with your friends. That gives you an accountability partner, and moving together makes it feel like less work.

SG: Is sex exercise?

JH: It is.

SG: Put it on the list.

JH: It is! There's even research showing how many calories it burns. It's a physical activity.

With so many good reasons to get moving, what are we waiting for? And please don't get hung up on the idea that you need to sweat profusely and find a budget to join a gym. You don't have to spend a lot of money to be active. A good pair of shoes and the right clothes for the weather are important if you're planning to walk, jog, or climb, but aside from that, the world is waiting for you—and a lot of it is free. You can walk on your own street or in a nearby green space. You can climb the stairs at work or in a mall. And community centres often have good programs for all ages and fitness levels. If some types of movement are difficult for you, don't be discouraged. There is always a way. All body sizes and shapes can find a suitable type of gentle or more demanding physical exercise. Yoga can be practised on a chair. Aquafit is a good option for those with joint pain. Some stretches can even be done in bed! The key is to make a commitment to moving more. Your body *and* your brain will thank you. If you move, you'll be moved.

Eat Well

Here comes another confession. Most of the time I eat well and clean, but I also enjoy some less healthy food once in a while. These days, I'll occasionally treat myself to a good poutine or a BeaverTail. I truly believe that "everything in moderation" is a good motto for eating and living.

If we're going to take care of our minds and move our bodies, we need to make sure we're nourishing them properly—and that means getting comfy in our kitchens. I don't know about you, but I practically live in mine—preparing meals, doing dishes, arguing, laughing, crying, dancing, sharing a glass of wine and chatting away with my mom or girlfriends. Our kitchen has seen so much, and it truly is the heart of our home.

If you walk into our kitchen, this is what you'll see: pictures on all the walls and stuck to the fridge with magnets. Speaking of magnets, we have quite the collection. "It's all shits and giggles until somebody giggles and shits," says one. Mae West offers: "You only live once, but if you do it well, once is enough." Leonard Cohen is there, too: "There's a crack in everything. That's where the light gets in." One of my favourites is from Robin Williams: "You're only given one little spark of madness. You mustn't lose it." (Wishing we hadn't lost him, and may his soul rest in peace.)

Once you stop reading the magnets, you'll probably notice Hadrien's toys and books lying in a corner, candles (always!) on the table, a double row of vitamins and some of my reading material on the counter, the kids' school and activities schedules taped on the wall, piles of work papers in one corner, and a shelf filled with crayons, colouring books, and kids' drawings. Oh, and there's also an old string of tiny white Christmas lights that I never took down, because they are magical.

And, of course, because this is the place where our family meals are prepared and eaten, there's food. As an adult, I'm grateful for the healthy eating habits my parents established when I was young. I was brought up on nutritious food (except for Cap'n Crunch cereal, which I was allowed to have on weekends and which I ate till it hurt the inside of my mouth). My mom would bring me to "the golden arches" once in a while, but that never seemed to work out well for me. My taste buds loved it, but my belly didn't, and I'd often find myself with an upset stomach afterwards.

Because I was so active as a child and teen, I became naturally curious about nutrition. I could feel the difference in my body when I nourished it with good food, and I also sensed how lethargic and bloated I could become if I ingested things that weren't as good for me. As the years went by, I became more interested in the links between gut health and brain health. I've learned that what we eat and how we eat is important; in fact, it affects the whole wheel of our well-being. In general, experts tell us, we eat too much and too fast.

Speaking about children, Dr. Bonnie J. Kaplan has noted that they "look well fed, they're always putting stuff in their mouths, but their brains are starving." Bonnie knows her stuff. She's professor emeritus in the Cumming School of Medicine at the University of Calgary. In 2017, she was selected as one of 150 Canadian Difference Makers in Mental Health, and in 2021, she was named one of the Top 7 Over 70 in Calgary. This recognition is partly due to her book *The Better Brain*, written with Julia Rucklidge, and partly due to her two charitable funds that support research by junior colleagues who study nutrition and mental health.

Dr. Kaplan is one of many scientists who have proven the importance of nutrition for mental health, and her primary goal is to bring nutrition education and treatment to the forefront of mental health care. It is, she explains, why she has chosen to do what she does. "I have seen this tremendous growth in information about what nutrients do in the brain and how important they are for brain health, and the general public doesn't know it," she told me. "Our book is written for the general public, not for scientific colleagues, and we really want everyone to understand and feel empowered. Empowered means that we can influence our own brain health so much, based on what we choose to put in our mouths." Although this interview is quite technical, it equipped me with an up-to-date understanding about nutrition that can be truly life-changing. Here we go:

Sophie Grégoire: Can you talk to us about the importance of vitamins and minerals to our brain?

Dr. Bonnie Kaplan: Nutrients such as minerals and vitamins create our brains, but I wonder if you've ever stopped and thought about the definition of *food*. Food is what we ingest in order to build and maintain our cellular activity. So that's exactly what good food does: it builds our cells and enables them to function. And if it's real food, then it provides the cofactors required for all of metabolism, but especially in the brain.

SG: What are *cofactors*?

BK: They do *everything* in the brain. If I had my way, the term *cofactor* would be explained starting in about grade six. It certainly should be taught in medical schools, and, frankly, it still isn't. A cofactor is a set of molecules that relies upon vitamins and minerals, which enable enzymatic reactions to happen.

Enzymes cannot do their work of transforming chemical A to chemical B if they do not have a continuous, abundant supply of vitamins and minerals for their cofactors. And those cofactors determine the rate at which those metabolic, energy-creating steps happen. Don't think of metabolic steps as happening or not happening; think of them as happening optimally or being rather feeble.

Sophie, it's amazing. Those of us who study broad-spectrum micronutrients select people in our studies for a disorder—say major depression or ADHD. But we aren't studying those things specifically; we're studying impulsivity and inattention and so forth. And we can say ADHD is especially a prefrontal lobe executive function deficit, but there's all kinds of mood dys-regulation stuff that goes along with it. So that's why when micronutrients work, there is across-the-board improvement.

SG: Now, what are *broad-spectrum micronutrients*?

BK: Most of us use the word *micronutrients* to mean vitamins and minerals. Essential fatty acids, amino acids, etc., they're all important, too, but the micronutrients are the cofactors. There are roughly fifteen vitamins and fifteen minerals.

SG: So let's simplify this. When I hear "fifteen vitamins and fifteen minerals," it's like, "Ahh! How do I get all those?" What does this look like in everyday life?

BK: It looks like eating real food, first of all. Don't eat the stuff inside the packaged goods—that's not doing you any good at all.

So we usually talk about a Mediterranean style of diet. And fill half your plate with fruits and vegetables. Nuts and seeds for your snacks. Olive oil, when possible. If you're not a vegetarian, eat fish a couple times a week, meat, dairy, eggs of a healthy kind. Data shows that so many kids are putting a lot of food in their mouths, but when you eat ultra-processed food, you are replacing the opportunity to feed your brain and you're harming your brain. It's not so much that it's high in calories, but it's devoid of the micronutrients that our brains need. And almost a quarter of your blood supply is feeding your brain every minute that your heart is beating, and if you're not feeding that source for your brain cells all the time, you're cheating your brain. Addiction to sugar and metabolic problems are real.

I'm old enough to remember when I suddenly realized that people were treating food as a treat. Our grandparents would be shocked. They ate to sustain their health, to be robust, to be healthy. Everybody knew nutrition was the foundation of resilience. There is no contradiction between this information and everything else you're covering [in terms of mental health benefits], from mindfulness, exercise, breathing—these are all very valuable. But if your brain is not working optimally, start with the foundation.

SG: Digestion issues are rampant. Is a good balance of prebiotics—leeks, garlic, onions, Jerusalem artichokes, and bananas, for example—mixed with probiotics—kimchi, kombucha, fermented foods, yogurt—a good formula to optimize gut health and therefore brain health?

BK: Yes. Go for the naturally occurring prebiotics and probiotics first, without a doubt.

SG: Serotonin, dopamine—can we talk about the feel-good hormones and how we need them for our mental well-being, and how nutrition and these hormones are linked? Is it because the enzymes need the micronutrients and the cofactors to be able to produce the hormones that affect mood?

BK: That's right. Our brain is only 2 percent of our body weight on average, so you would think that our brain would suck up 2 percent of the nutrients that we eat and you'd be wrong. Because even at rest, our brains are pulling in at least ten times that proportion of micronutrients, because it is the most metabolically active organ that we have.

So, when you eat, you really are eating primarily for your brain—there is no question about that. I don't know how to make serotonin, but my brain can do it through the food I feed my gut. And all I need to do is give it the building blocks, and those are primarily vitamins and minerals and omega-3s that are very important for cell walls, etc. That's why we need to be eating those whole foods, and that's why we need our farmers to improve the mineral content of our soil.

SG: What are *mitochondria?*

BK: Oh, the mitochondria are just fascinating. Humans have them in every single cell in our brain and body, and some cells have dozens and dozens of them. And what they do is produce ATP—the energy molecule. If you don't have ATP, you're not alive.

And that, by the way, is very relevant to gut function, and a lot of people don't realize this. One of the things that ATP does is balance inflammation. Now, inflammation is not all bad. Inflammatory responses are really good when you're trying to fight off a virus, but excessive inflammation caused by a bad diet is really bad. We shouldn't be looking at anti-inflammatory drugs all the time; we should be improving our production of ATP, because that is the way to fight inflammation. ATP sucks that up. It all comes back to nutrition, really.

There are sixty to seventy studies worldwide showing that micronutrients should be a major treatment for mental health problems, and nutrition education should be part of every prevention program. We've been trying to teach people to eat better for fifty years, and teaching them to cook. But until we teach them why it matters, I don't think we'll see much behaviour change. If we teach people why they need to feed their brains every minute of every day, when they learn about what nutrients do in those metabolic pathways, it changes how they select their food. So that's what I'd like to leave people with.

Get Some Sleep!

Tell me, how do you sleep? I was always a great sleeper, but my thirties and forties have been peppered with sleep disturbances.

Having babies meant many sleepless nights, and I became a very light sleeper who wakes at the tiniest sound. Sleepy teas, fans, ear plugs, meditation, and extra pillows: I've tried them all! What about you? Are you an early bird or a night owl? How many hours do you get and how deep do you go? Whatever your pattern, the truth is that humans function better biologically after proper rest. I know so many people who have worked night shifts at some point during their career (myself included), and the anecdotal evidence suggests that it really throws you off in ways you didn't expect. We are not meant to live on little sleep, and science is now showing us how sleep is paramount for good mental health.

I've always been an early riser. My dad, with his mischievous nature, would walk into my room at around six in the morning on weekends and blow his hand-held boat horn and shout, "Soph! The lake is like a mirror! Let's go water-skiing!" I was often mad about the rude awakening, but I couldn't resist a calm lake. I knew how incredible it was to skim the water at that time and how refreshed I would feel after.

I can still picture my own alarm clock (no blaring horns there) set to 6:45 a.m. for pretty much all of my teenage years. That was the time I woke up in order to get ready for school, have a quick breakfast, and walk to catch the 7:45 a.m. city bus. Now, as a mom of two teenagers, I realize that I might have been unusual in my desire to get up and at it every day. My kids seem to want to go to bed later and wake up later. I know it's part of their altered circadian rhythm as they go through adolescence, but I still try to encourage them to not hit the pillow too late. I've read that if it takes you less than five minutes to fall asleep at night, it probably means you are overtired. (It usually takes Justin a whole three minutes! Welcome to the life of a prime minister.)

I get really grumpy when I haven't slept well. Science shows that a lack of good sleep can affect our energy level, our mood, our focus, our hunger, our patience, our sociability, our anxiety, our stress levels, and our capacity for perspective in our decision-making. It can also lead to emotional exhaustion, which can make us increasingly irritable. Dr. Amy Wheeler, CEO and director of Optimal State—an organization dedicated to training health-care practitioners to provide embodied mental health care to individuals experiencing burnout, insomnia, anxiety, depression, chronic pain, and stress—explained why this happens. "According to the Ayurvedic clock, the hippocampus is an area in the brain that sorts our memories from the day, and that happens from ten p.m. to two a.m.," she told me. "So, if we miss that window of sleep, we miss the memory sorting for the day, and it's almost like not taking the trash out of your mind, you know? So, if you go to bed at one a.m. and wake up at nine a.m., that's a very different eight hours of sleep than going to bed from nine p.m. to five a.m."

In a sleep study led by the Canadian Mental Health Association, lead author Dr. Michael Wainberg wrote, "The relationship between sleep and mental health is bi-directional. Poor sleep contributes to poor mental health and poor mental health contributes to poor sleep." More than 30 percent of Canadians suffer from insomnia, and millions of others have disturbed sleep patterns. Too many kids and teenagers are also sleep-deprived. Combined with a nutritious lunch, sleep is the most essential school supply for our kids. And whether we're talking about kids or adults, the formula is the same: mix lack of sleep with lack of exercise and bad nutrition and you've got a recipe for trouble. We become overtired. Nervous fatigue sets in. We feel "off" most of the time. It's so difficult to perform, be creative, and sustain a positive outlook on life when you don't get enough sleep. And we also know that sleep problems are common in those with mental health issues like anxiety, depression, or ADHD. The good news is that creating better sleep habits is within our control. We can build a "better sleep toolbox" to dip into when we find ourselves struggling to get a good night's rest.

If we're worried about getting enough sleep, one of the tools in that box may seem counterintuitive: stop worrying. Of course, we all have things we're concerned about and that require careful thought. But constant worrying can turn into a negative mental habit, which in turn can affect our sleep. Dr. Judson Brewer, psychiatrist and author of *Unwinding Anxiety*, explains that "worrying is activating, and as we get worried, our energy ramps up," making it difficult to nod off. "And then we start worrying that we can't get to sleep and we're not going to get enough sleep. And so that just feeds on itself, especially if we look at the clock or look at our phone and realize that we've been worrying for two hours and we're nowhere any closer to sleep."

When that happens, Dr. Brewer tells us, we can look to curiosity for help. "If we're truly curious about our own minds, we can learn to step out of our old habits," he says. So, if worries (about sleep or anything else) are stopping us from getting the rest we need, we can rob them of their power by asking questions instead of getting stuck in a spin cycle. Why am I worrying if I am safe in this present moment? Is this something I can control? If no, why am I worrying about it? If yes, then what good is worrying about it now going to do? Is there a better time and place to think about this issue?

If you've tried asking yourself these questions and still aren't able to quiet your mind, consider incorporating a mindfulness practice during the day or before going to bed (for more on mindfulness, see chapter 9). A simple body scan can be a good way to start. Quietly observe each part of your body, starting with the top of your head and moving to the bottom of your feet, and softly focus on what's happening and how you feel. Eventually, you'll be able to quiet your mind, which will let you quiet your body. Once this happens, falling asleep comes more easily.

Another tool in that better sleep toolbox came up during my conversation with Jennifer Heisz. She told me that the amount we move and exercise during the day has a direct impact on the quality of our sleep at night. "The body produces a natural sleep aid called adenosine," she explained. "Now, the cool thing about adenosine is that it's the by-product of the breakdown of our energy currency. So our cells have this energy currency they use called ATP. When we expend that energy, it produces adenosine. So, when we move more during the day, we're using more ATP and we're producing more adenosine."

My Better Sleep Toolbox

Over the years, I've found a few things that help me settle down for a good night's sleep. Maybe some of them will work for you, too.

- Avoid eating for at least two hours before bed (if you must eat something, try a light snack like a banana or almonds).
- Avoid excessive exercise for at least two hours before bed.
- Limit alcohol intake before bed (and throughout the day).
- Make time to journal, writing down any worrying thoughts and your to-do list for the next day.
- Make sure your brain feels safe as you get ready for slumber.
- Turn off all electronic devices, preferably sixty minutes before bed (start with thirty minutes and see the difference).
- Try to go for a walk outdoors near the end of the day.
- Take a warm bath (but not too hot, as that can activate energy levels).
- Turn your room into a haven (light a candle, spray your sheets with a calming diluted essential oil).
- Practise five to twenty minutes of yoga nidra. Yoga nidra is a guided meditation that brings you to a state between waking and sleeping. There are many options available online.
- Try yin yoga and restorative yoga. Yin is a slow and relaxing pace of yoga that incorporates principles of traditional Chinese medicine. In yin yoga, postures (asanas) are held for longer periods than in other styles. Restorative yoga is similar to yin but typically uses the support of props such as bolsters, blankets, or eye pillows. It is mood-enhancing and helps shift the balance from the sympathetic nervous system (freeze-fight-flight) to the parasympathetic nervous system (relaxation response).
- Try tapping (also known as EFT, or emotional freedom techniques). Tapping is a simple relaxation technique based on

the combined principles of ancient Chinese acupressure points and modern psychology. It is used to treat symptoms of anxiety, pain, headaches, depression, and more. It's not time-consuming, and you can teach it to yourself. Search "tapping" or "EFT" online to find out more.

NOTE: These tips are helpful ways to allow your nervous system to relax, but they are not meant to heal deep psychological distress. If you are ready and/or interested in addressing some of your core issues, know that there are tools out there for you such as cognitive behavioural therapy, psychoanalysis, psychiatry, EMDR (eye movement desensitization and reprocessing), and many other approaches to fit your needs. Don't hesitate to ask for help!

Our bodies are so naturally wise, aren't they? When we eat well, we can move more. And when we move more, we can better manage stress and anxiety and sleep. And when we sleep better, we're able to be our best selves in terms of job performance, creativity, relationships, and so much more. The body is truly an intuitive machine. If we pay attention, we realize that it often speaks directly to us, expressing what the mind has tried to suppress and telling us exactly what we need. The more in tune we are with it, the better able we are to dial into and foster that wisdom.

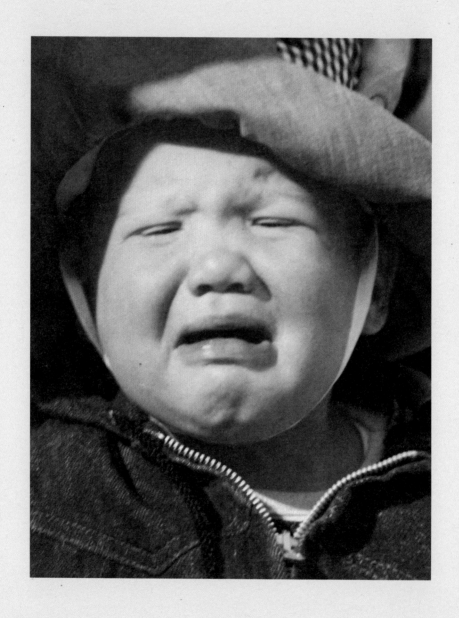

The Two Wolves

Tackling the Tough Stuff and Coming Out on Top

Paradoxically, the more we're willing to be
uncomfortable, the more ease we'll find.

SETH GILLIHAN

It's a cold January morning and I've been up since five thirty. Didi often comes into bed with me and he wiggles—a lot—so I've been tossing and turning for a while. I read him a short story at around six thirty, boil water for a quick cup of tea, and jump into my car to drive myself and Ella-Grace to a medical appointment. We register at reception and then sit and wait for our names to be called. The place is already half-full and it just opened. Ella and I are whisper-chatting and reading when a man enters the room, breathing loudly and addressing the receptionist in a voice to match: "Yeah," he says angrily, as everyone looks on, "I'm here because of my cold, the Trudeau cold!"

My daughter turns to me in disbelief and lifts her eyes to the sky. We exchange a sigh and a smile—we've been through this before—but inside I'm ready to pounce. The blood vessels in my face dilate, my heart beats faster, and my gut roils. I want to protect my family and tell this angry man that he's got it all wrong, but I won't, of course. Instead, I try to notice my rising emotions, understand them, and reassure myself. At the same time, I continue to pay attention to everything the man is saying. I try to dig into my capacity for compassion. Another part of me would love to just sit with him, listen to him, make him laugh, and maybe find something we have in common—like a love for animals or motorbikes. And then I'd introduce myself so he might have a better idea of my humanity.

Allowing ourselves to notice and then feel our emotions in challenging moments like this isn't easy, but it's so necessary. "Violence is what happens when we don't know what else to do with our suffering," says author Parker J. Palmer.

To suppress any of our emotions—sadness, anger, rage, depression—is a sure-fire way to experience more of the same and to risk repercussions in our capacity to have healthy relationships with others and ourselves. What is felt needs to be expressed in order to progress— even if what is felt isn't so great. Recently, I watched the TV series *Limitless*, featuring Chris Hemsworth. In a discussion about how to control our emotions and anxiety, psychologist Modupe Akinola said that we need to "date our stress." What she meant is that we need to embrace it, get comfortable with it, and face it head on in order to overcome it. The same holds true for all of our negative emotions. We also need to recognize that the mindset with which we approach our own difficult emotions will affect the outcome. In *A Year of Miracles*, author and spiritual leader Marianne Williamson writes, "It is our own thoughts that hold the key to miraculous transformation. Negativity poisons my mind, and positivity restores it. A moment of crisis can be a moment of growth, as the wounded self prepares to transform."

These are words to hold close as we confront the little and big challenges of our own lives. Everyone on this planet will face obstacles

206

at some point or another, regardless of cultural, social, religious, or economic background.

I can reflect on my own past and see how easy it would have been for difficult times (including the loss of a very young cousin to a "hanging game" just before I entered my teen years) to have derailed me and some of the people I love dearly. I'm sure you have difficult times of your own. Maybe you grew up in a dysfunctional family or a marginalized community. Maybe you suffer from an addiction, or are trying to make ends meet as a single parent. Maybe you are a teen being bullied at school, or a young adult struggling to find your place in the world. The size of the obstacle doesn't matter; it's part of being human, part of being alive in this world. What matters is how we choose to deal with the fallout, with the negative thoughts and behaviours that can all too easily take over and hold us back. The good news is that we all have the power to adjust our mindset and break our negative patterns. We can become more flexible psychologically, and boldly open ourselves up to feeling whatever must be felt without shame or guilt.

It all comes down to which patterns we choose to nourish. Have you ever heard the Cherokee story about the two wolves? "I have a fight going on in me," a grandfather told his grandson. "It's taking place between two wolves. One is evil—he is anger, envy, sorrow, regret, greed, arrogance, self-pity, guilt, resentment, inferiority, lies, false pride, superiority, and ego." The grandfather looked at his grandson and went on. "The other embodies positive emotions. He is joy, peace, love, hope, serenity, humility, kindness, benevolence, empathy, generosity, truth, compassion, and faith. Both wolves are fighting to their death. The same fight is going on inside you and every other person, too." The grandson took a moment to reflect. At last, he looked up at his grandfather and asked, "Which wolf will win?" The old man gave a simple reply: "The one you feed."

This parable serves as a powerful reminder that we can't let ourselves be beaten down by the things that happen to us. We get to choose how to react to those experiences. We can turn them to our advantage by integrating the lessons they teach. We can conquer the "evil wolf" inside our own mind by purposefully turning toward the light instead of the darkness, every time. Later in this chapter, we'll talk more about how we can do this, but first, let's talk more about some of those evil wolves.

Riding the Wave of Fear

The Buddhist nun and author Pema Chödrön teaches us that "to be fully alive, fully human, and completely awake is to be continually thrown out of the nest . . . nothing ever goes away until it has taught us what we need to know. Nothing ever really attacks us except our own confusion . . . Fear brings us closer to the truth."

Sometimes our darkest moments, filled with uncertainty and a sense of abandonment, are the ones from which we can learn the most. Rarely do we feel an intense negative emotion that does not have fear at its base. At one point or another, we're all afraid. It's a core part of the human experience, hard-wired into our brains to help us identify threats. Brené Brown says, "People buy into [fear] and feel fear because they don't have the language to attach to what it is. It implies anxiety and lack of courage."

What is your relationship with fear? From personal experience as well as conversations with experts, I've learned that fear is the most mobilizing *and* immobilizing state we can be in. It can keep us from harm and propel us into action, but it can also lock us in a state of toxic alertness. Fear and anxiety are best buddies, but they are not *our* friends. And although we know deep down inside that these emotions can pass, that can be hard to remember in moments when they seem to have a firm grip on the wheel.

I was never really fearful as a girl or teenager, and I wouldn't say I'm fearful now, as a grown woman. In fact, those who know me well might say that I'm quite courageous. But over the last few years, that courage has been tested in many ways, and I've had to look fear full in the face.

To help me do that, and to stop fear from taking over, I often imagine it as a wave. The highest literal wave I've ever surfed—about eight feet—was in Tofino, British Columbia, in 2018. It was a very foggy and windy day, so visibility was awful. Just swimming to the break was a feat. I got pounded and thumped by the water and was kept under for so long that there were moments when I honestly thought I wasn't going to make it back to the surface. Every time I managed to catch a breath of air, it literally felt as if I were coming back to life.

To become a good surfer, you must be a very strong swimmer, be physically fit, and understand the tides, winds, and wave patterns. When you're on your board and you see a wave or a set of waves coming your way, you must determine whether the wave will crash, die down, or lift so you can surf it properly. Once you've figured out if it's going to naturally take you left or right, you position yourself on your board, start paddling, continue to look at it from both sides, and then paddle with everything you've got so you can try to match its speed. The second you feel that lift, it's time to pop up—light as a feather—and drop to surf it. For about a millisecond, there is a feeling of weightlessness, and then comes the speed of descent. It's exhilarating. If your breathing is too erratic and you're not relaxed enough, you might miss the momentum. But if your observation, body placement, attitude, and breath are all accurate and in synch, you might just catch the wave of your life. And then the next.

So how is surfing a wave in the ocean similar to surfing the wave of fear? Like an ocean wave, fear usually comes and goes. There is also a discernible pattern to how it shows up and what creates or triggers it. Think about what those triggers are for you. Financial uncertainty? Rejection? Loneliness? Apart from situations in which there is an imminent danger to your physical or psychological safety—in which case fear is warranted and necessary—fear usually shows up when you are projecting yourself into an unknown future. It's as if you're imagining a worst-case scenario every time, and it's so draining that the delusion about that future almost becomes your present. If you've ever had a panic attack, you know what this feels like. You are locked in alert mode, convinced you're about to go into cardiac arrest, maybe even die, because of the pressure you feel in your chest, for example. Your thoughts are running wild and your mind is feeding your physical symptoms, which are just getting worse and worse. But really, you're not dying, and this will pass. It's just hard to see that in the moment.

Have you ever felt like this? I certainly have. Only now, at forty-eight years old, I can see the wave coming. I can observe myself slipping into a fearful state of mind. I feel the fear like a wave heading toward me, and I try my best to watch it and contemplate it in the same way I might watch an ocean wave I'm thinking of riding but haven't yet committed to. How can I best catch that wave? What should my emotional posture be? How will I slow down my breathing amid the noise and get ready to become lighter, safe in the knowledge that fear, just like a wave, will pass, and there is always a horizon beyond the waves? Sometimes, the wave that almost breaks you can also be the one that builds you as it becomes the ride of your life.

I haven't always been successful when it comes to pushing fear away or observing that wave. There have been many times I've felt vulnerable, exposed, and unsafe. On one awful day in 2014, I had recently given birth, Justin was away, and the kids, a girlfriend, and I were sleeping upstairs. In the morning, we discovered that an intruder had broken into our home and left a note by the back door with knives all around it. On several occasions, protesters have tried to physically harm Justin as we've walked in a parade as a family. Our family has been told, at the last minute, not to join him on stage during a political rally because of imminent threats, and all of us have body-guards 24/7, at work, school, and play. My children have seen posters of their dad standing on the gallows in front of an executioner, and we've seen "F✿ck Trudeau" signs in car and truck windows while walking or driving around town.

It's hard to experience and see things like this and not react. It's hard to accept that threats, bullying, and uneasiness are part of your day-to-day life, and it's hard, as a parent, to think that your kids might not be or feel secure in the midst of all this. It puts your mind in a constant state of high alert that can be difficult to manage. Some days, it takes everything I have to not let fear consume me while my amygdala keeps ringing the bell of distress. But I keep working at it, no matter what my brain is telling me in the moment. I want to train my brain to come back into safety mode every time.

The Ability to Respond

Riding the wave of fear is something we can all aspire to, but it's never easy. In this particular era, where everything is polarized and where hateful thoughts and words can be put out into the world with a few keystrokes, it's hard to stay on top of that wave, or even to observe it with a critical, dispassionate eye. It's hard to keep fear, anxiety, stress, depression, or any other negative thought patterns or behaviours at bay. And it's especially hard to figure out how best to deal with the small-t and big-T traumas that we may have accumulated during our years on the planet. But it helps to remember that we are still in charge. We are the ones who get to decide how to deal with our emotions.

Basically, we have two choices. Either we settle into a "victim consciousness," where we constantly blame others and life circumstances for our unhappiness and lack of control, or we choose to live from an "empowered consciousness," where we take responsibility for and control of our thoughts and actions. As Dr. Gabor Maté told me, there is no consciousness without responsibility. "When people say 'I'm a survivor,' they're identifying with a particular experience. But they're much more than that experience. And so, when people identify with a victim role, they're actually limiting themselves."

He went on to explain that trauma is not what happened to you. "'What happened to you?' is an important question," he says, "but what happened to you is not who you are. And trauma is not what happened to you; trauma is what happened inside you as a result of what happened to you. Trauma is the wound. So, when you say, 'I'm a victim,' you're saying, 'I'm wounded.' But you're not *just* wounded—you're also somebody with the capacity for healing."

When we identify only with the wounded part of ourselves, Dr. Maté says, we are limiting who we are and not taking responsibility. "By responsibility, I don't mean blame—you're not to be blamed for what happened, but only you, in the present moment, can be responsible for how you deal with it. So to give up the victim stance is to embrace responsibility—not guilt, not blame—responsibility, the ability to respond."

Dr. Maté's words feel especially relevant in our current culture. After our discussion, I found myself wondering how much of what we're dealing with these days—from a toxic online culture to intolerance to polarized debates on almost any topic you can think of—is the result of an inability or unwillingness to respond to challenges with an open and clear mind. And if this is the case, how and where did we lose this ability? Is it possible that our minds have become too set in their ways, too comfortable with what is familiar, too "fixed" in constant loops of negativity and fear? What would happen if we felt safe enough to gain perspective on our thought patterns, and to be conscious of when we are caught in a pit of negativity and fear? What would happen if we had tools that we could use to make our brains more "flexible" and able to adapt to life's challenges with more predictability and less uncertainty?

A fixed mind is a dangerous mind. It can distort the truth to fit its own comfort or discomfort zones, and can become a living and powerful threat not only to our emotional well-being but also to the world at large. A fixed mind is harsh, fearful, aggressive, conspiracy-driven. It is eagerly looking for friends to share feelings of anger with. True freedom, and true humanity, lies in a liberated mind—but how do we get there? How do we overcome past traumas, negative thought patterns, and whatever else plagues us, to approach the world from a healthier, happier place? How do we stop feeding those bad wolves and start nourishing the good ones?

Dr. David Livingstone Smith is a professor of philosophy at the University of New England and the author of several books, including *On Inhumanity* and *Making Monsters*. He's thought a lot about the dangerous implications of a fixed mind and about how we can work to become more flexible. I gained so much insight from what he shared.

Sophie Grégoire: You've stated, in your work, that you want to address the brokenness of the human condition. Are we truly broken?

Dr. David Livingstone Smith: Well, I think our true nature is complicated, that we have sides we approve of and sides we disapprove of. And we're embedded in a social world with lots of pressures on us. So human beings, I think, are massive contradictions. It's hard because we'd like to simplify ourselves and distill ourselves down to something nice, but that's unrealistic. And I think a lot of misery comes through the difficulty acknowledging the complexity and contradictoriness of the human condition.

There are two sides to understanding dehumanization. One thing is what's in our heads, and the other is what our heads are in. That's the social and political environment, and to understand dehumanization, you need to take both of these things into account. Normalcy is really a con.

SG: So, what is *dehumanization*? Racism, transphobia. What else?

DLS: The way I use the term *dehumanization*—and people use it in wildly different ways—is thinking of others as subhuman creatures. Nearby phenomena are things like ordinary racism, although dehumanization and racism are very intimately connected. Sexism is a nearby phenomenon. Transphobia, ableism, those nasty "isms." And the reason I like to make the distinction between dehumanization in a narrow sense and these other things is because I think all of these things have their unique dynamics. We can only intervene properly if we understand the dynamics of each.

SG: Depression, blame, and paranoia—you say those are the three culprits that perpetrators use to actually lure people and make them feel vulnerable. So, for example, making people feel depressed about their lives, pointing the finger at other people as the reason for their depressed state, and then making them feel like the world or a group of people is conspiring against them in a way?

DLS: Exactly. This kind of propaganda only works because it's around in the culture and it's meant to manipulate. It's sort of sedimented in and it's easily ignited. And people in positions of influence can light that match and put it to that dry kindling and—bang! That can be very, very difficult to resist.

SG: So we are urgently called to develop our capacity for discernment and get out of our fixed mindsets?

DLS: Oh yeah, absolutely. We need to help young people to be courageous, imaginative, critical thinkers. You have to be able to place yourself in the situation of others.

SG: In order to develop our capacity for discernment, we first need to be independent thinkers?

DLS: Exactly. And that's subversive, you see, because that allows people to resist the forces pressing in on them that want to shape them in certain ways.

SG: In your most recent book, *Making Monsters*, you say that under hate lies a longing for connection. Please tell us more.

DLS: Here I agree with Plato, reporting on Socrates—the idea that we're always seeking the good. We are just ignorant of what the good is. People pursue what they think is best. Unfortunately, that's not a straightforward thing. So the horrible things that people do to one another, there is a longing behind that. They're trying to make their lives and even the lives of others better in a very misguided way. They're not there cackling and going, "I want to do evil." They really think that this awful stuff is going to save the world. But I think there is, to use a term that I don't use very often, a positive impulse at the heart of a lot of this awful, evil stuff.

SG: Are there a lot of repressed emotions in individuals who have been the perpetrators of divisiveness, hate, disgust, repulsion?

DLS: Sure, sure, absolutely. But I think there's a place for all of these emotions. It's to the right degree at the right time. There's certainly room for despair, rage, righteous anger, guilt, or shame, but it has to be fitting. Because of the work I do, I fairly often encounter pretty unpleasant people. I certainly try to not shame them. We've got to keep our eyes on the prize here. If we want to facilitate change in a positive direction, we need to be curious and compassionate and engage in genuine conversations with people. Some won't play ball, but even then, I think a significant number will come away from a conversation like that with some seeds of doubt planted. We all want to be loved. We all want to be respected and at peace.

We have that innate recognition of the humanness of one another. And that innate recognition encourages us to treat others with decency and with respect. And that gives me hope. We've got to push back against those forces that want to fragment us, that want to exploit us, but not by dehumanizing them, too. All those negative emotions have to be respected in a way as they interrogate you.

What David is telling us is that, as with so much in life, compassion is key. We must challenge ourselves, daily, to be more compassionate, especially when it's hard. Are we generally accepting of ourselves and others, or only when we feel like being kind? There's a big difference. Offering compassion means seeing yourself and the other in the truest light and not being threatened. Rose-Marie Charest put it so well: "[T]he more fragile we are, the more intolerant we are of difference. It's true in families and it's true in society." I believe tolerance alone is not enough, as it implies conditions; what we must strive for is acceptance and respect. To be filled with respect for others means opening our minds and our hearts. In the face of difficulty, acceptance and compassion is understanding one's suffering. In the face of happiness and positivity, it is feeling a shared joy for someone else's success and well-being. This kind of compassion can transform into an attitude of love and kindness. And this is the prize we must keep our eye on.

Rising Above

No matter what you've had to face or endure in your life, it is worth holding on to what both Dr. Smith and Dr. Maté have shared with us. Compassion is key—for ourselves and others. And we get to choose how to respond to the events in our lives. Remind yourself that you can do this in a way that will empower and build rather than weaken and destroy. You can feed the good wolf instead of the evil one. This is where our power lies: we can choose to deal with our negative patterns and emotions in ways that don't lock us in but instead allow us to become freer thinkers and feelers.

As author Viktor Frankl wrote in *Man's Search for Meaning*: "When we can no longer change a situation, we are challenged to change ourselves." Frankl, who survived the horrors of concentration camps, wrote that those around him who had a rich spiritual life usually had more resilience and psychological flexibility to sustain themselves through the unsustainable.

My friend Jewel Kilcher has exhibited tremendous resilience and psychological flexibility in a life that has featured its fair share of challenges. Her father was an alcoholic who was badly abused as a child, and as Jewel once said in an interview with the *New York Times*, "Hurt people hurt people. We want to villainize it, but it's always somebody hurt that's hurting someone." For a time, she lived in her van, and ended up in a mental spiral that could have had devastating consequences. Fortunately, Jewel decided to change her life—and change her brain at the same time.

Two decades ago, she created the Inspiring Children Foundation, a non-profit dedicated to helping youth development in underserved communities. She believes that therapy, support, forgiveness, and gratitude go a long way when it comes to healing. As she put it in one of her poems, "We are not in the business of fighting darkness, we are farmers of light."

What Jewel's personal story shows us is that in order to break out of negative emotion and thought patterns, we must figure out how to deal with pain. We must learn how to quiet the noise, how to survive and adapt, how to step away from our distractions and fall safely into the intimacy of presence. Meet Jewel. Hear about her quest to understand herself better and her wise insight on how to help others who struggle.

Sophie Grégoire: Your foundation works with struggling youth. What are you learning about them?

Jewel Kilcher: What I've seen is that as a society, we forgot what to do with pain. We're supposed to deal with pain. Our stress system is like an immune system. It gets stronger the more stress it gets to experience. But just like an immune system, if you have an overwhelming illness, your body can tank. So the trick with your immune system is giving it stimulation at healthy and appropriate times to build your immune response. Same with our stress system. Kids' brains are being flooded with images quicker than the brain can process, and that's causing cortisol levels to rise and creating an addiction to their own neural chemistry, which is excitatory, to the point where they think that the calming neurochemicals are boring. It's a heck of a pickle we've gotten ourselves into. We're talking about a depleted cultural soil when it comes to emotional intelligence and emotional adaptability.

SG: Is all this pain more imaginary than real in how it's processed by the brain?

JK: Yes. It's an over-identification with your thoughts, with your judgments of yourself. Emotional impermanence is real. If you look at the universe, it culminates in change. Whatever bad feeling you're having now, it can't last forever. And so, what I teach my kids is, you buckle yourself in and you know it will pass, as intense as it is, and then you go try and figure out how to help that feeling change.

When we try to disassociate from negative parts of ourselves, it won't change, because nothing changes in isolation. We're seeing that as a country. We can't fractionalize ourselves. We have to be in relationship for things to change.

217

SG: Knowing this, how do you teach emotional literacy to youth?

JK: It's kind of a multi-pronged approach. One facet is to quiet the noise. Getting kids off their devices. We are so distracted we don't actually know what we're feeling or thinking in real time. We want to stop and have formed, thoughtful responses. Not just knee-jerk reactions.

The second phase is teaching the names of feelings. You're not actually angry; you're hungry. Or you're not actually angry; you're scared. Just helping kids identify and match the right name to the right internal stimulus is a huge part of it.

SG: What would be an antidote to distraction?

JK: Conscious presence. Mindfulness is being consciously present. So anything that builds the muscle of being consciously present. And it is a muscle. In eight weeks of meditating three times a day, you can build a new fold in your frontal lobe.

When I was eighteen, I was homeless. I was having bad panic attacks. I was agoraphobic and I was shoplifting a lot. And I knew that if I kept shoplifting, I'd probably end up in jail. So I knew I was in a really dangerous place. I never drank, I never did drugs, but I was fully addicted to stealing. I remember being in a dressing room trying to steal a dress. I was shoving this dress down my pants. And I was like, "Maybe I can turn my life around one thought at a time." But I couldn't witness what I was thinking in real time. I didn't know the word *disassociation*, but I was dissociative. And so I started realizing my hands were the servants of my thoughts. So, if I want to know what I'm thinking, watch what my hands are doing, because it's thought slowed down into action.

So, for three weeks, I followed my hands around, writing down everything they did. And at the end of three weeks, I figured I was going to see what I was thinking. It was the best life plan I could come up with.

At the end of the three weeks, I realized my panic attacks had gone away. I didn't even realize it in real time. It wasn't until I sat down three weeks later that I was like, "Wait a minute. I haven't had a panic attack during this whole thing. Why?" What I'd stumbled on to was conscious presence.

SG: And how did you build on that?

JK: The next thing was: "Okay, one of my biggest pain points is stealing. This is what's going to land me in the most trouble if I can't figure out how to stop." And so, now that I'd learned to cultivate a little bit of real-time awareness, I was trying to understand, basically, addiction.

I'd always kind of "wake up" after I'd stolen. That's why that moment in the mirror when I was shoving the dress down my pants was so shocking, because I usually wasn't aware during it. I was only aware after.

The very, very, very last thing that came was replacing the behaviour. So, stimulus I couldn't do a lot about. I was really stressed because I was homeless. My response was stealing. My reward was I felt powerful, in control; it was exciting; it was distracting. So I started to replace stealing with writing. I loved writing. I've written my whole life. But it didn't feel good. And that was so curious to me. Why didn't writing, which I love, feel as good as stealing? And that's where I really had to get in my body. And again, through a lot of curiosity and a lot of observation, I thought about stealing. My whole system, like, contracted. It was exciting. When I think about writing, I think about this [emulates a posture of freeing, letting go, not controlling]. And that was so interesting. Those are two different body postures. One was excitatory and contracted, and one was dilated and open.

So I started to write down in my notebook every time I noticed I was dilated, every time I noticed I was contracted. I did it for a month. And what I realized is, we only have these two states of being. Dilated and contracted. And every single thought, feeling, or action leads us into one of these two states.

Now, I didn't know when I was eighteen that this is actually your parasympathetic nervous system and your sympathetic nervous system. In an excitatory state, a contracted state, you have constricted, heightened blood pressure, and your blood flow is charging into your amygdala and the fight-or-flight parts of your brain. In a calmative state, a dilated vascular system sends blood flow into your frontal lobes.

I was addicted to a contracted state. And that made a lot of sense. I was raised in an intense and abusive household. I learned to perform well in a contracted, heightened, excited, scared, anxious state. That was my neurological home.

I believe that if you choose your inner landscape, your outer landscape changes. So I believe in coming at things from the inside out. Cultivating a relationship with yourself is the most powerful and transformative thing you can do. It's the best investment you'll make.

What is your neurological home, in the sense that Jewel describes? Do you remember which states you were mostly in during your own youth? Performance? Protection? Avoidance? Rage? A bit of all of that, or something entirely different? My emotional home featured joy, anger, things unsaid, warmth, obsession with appearances, compassion, courage, isolation, emotional instability, humour, wit, depression, and, of course, love. And I've carried so much of that with me into adulthood.

Jewel's story is inspiring. The fact that she was able to overcome the trauma of her youth and go on to accomplish all that she has shows that we really do have the ability to respond. And if we stop to look, we'll see that we are surrounded by people like her, people who have risen above challenges and gone on to great things. In Canada, you need look no further than our governor general.

Mary Simon is Canada's first Indigenous governor general. She was born in Kangiqsualujjuaq, Nunavik (Quebec), to Nancy May (née Angnatuk-Askew), her Inuk mother, and Bob Mardon May, her father, who'd moved to the Arctic to work for the Hudson's Bay Company. After growing up in Kuujjuaq, a small, isolated community, she went on to become a journalist. She became known internationally for her work on Indigenous and Arctic issues, and for her advocacy work in the areas of Inuit rights, youth, education, and culture. And then, when she turned forty, she suffered a depression so severe that she was unable to function.

When we talked, she told me about that difficult time in her life, and about her decision to speak publicly about her mental health journey.

Sophie Grégoire: What did depression feel like?

Mary Simon: Kind of like rock bottom, like burnout. A bunch of accumulated things were happening within me. And I couldn't function. I had to see a doctor two or three times a week. I got myself a psychologist. And I went to the psychologist for five years. But at the beginning, it was extremely hard to talk about what was going on in my body, in my head. And it was just letting my emotions out. Just crying and letting it happen was the first thing that I had to do. And that's what my doctor told me: "Let your emotions out. You know it's okay for you to cry." Because I was always trying to stop myself.

When I was in my early stages of recovering, I went through periods where I just lay down and couldn't do anything else because the pain was overwhelming. It didn't allow me to even think. And the only thought that was always in my head was "How do I get out of this pain?" And at times, it was a feeling of hopelessness, because even after taking my medication or going to the counsellor or the psychologist, the pain would still be there. So there were times when you just said to yourself, "Let's get rid of this. Let's get rid of this." It's an emptiness. There's no hope. It's hard to describe where the pain is. It must be throughout your body, but you don't really know where. You think it's in your heart. Or sometimes it's in your head. But it's a pain that I could never explain with another type of pain.

SG: Did your upbringing have an impact on your mental well-being?

MS: We were not traumatized at home, but we were traumatized outside of the home—for instance, when we were in federal day school. It was a small community. We had a certain group of friends, and we all stuck to each other. So we'd be walking to school and we'd be laughing and playing and speaking Inuktitut, and then, as we got closer to the school, we'd start whispering. And at one point, we'd tell each other, "Don't talk Inuktitut anymore," because we were punished for speaking our language in our community. We couldn't speak our language on school grounds or in school, so to me, that was a trauma, but we didn't explain that to our parents.

SG: When we are not afraid of what we've been through, we can share our story. What is it that you want people to learn from yours?

MS: I find because I'm so grounded in what I feel and what I went through, it stays with me all the time. It gives me a lot of strength, to not be afraid of it. I'm not afraid to talk about it because it's not a weakness. See, that's how it used to be—if you expressed any kind of depression or sadness, you were just a weak person. But it's the opposite. And we have to get people to understand that it's a strength to be able to acknowledge that, first, you're going through a difficult time, which is painful, and second, that you're trying to find ways of dealing with it and you need other people to help you. And we don't have a system that allows for that relationship to build and bond. For many, many years, the system has been focused on physical health. So, every time you break your arm or you have a headache or whatever, the doctor is there. But with mental health, first you have to convince them that you are going through something that's pretty bad, and then the structure doesn't support that. So people wait for months to try and see a counsellor. The number one challenge is to give mental health the same kind of importance and recognition as physical well-being. Because without mental health, your physical health goes to pot.

What Mary Simon and Jewel and so many others have learned, through their own struggles and accomplishments, is that we are capable of being in charge of our own lives. We can take the difficult things that life throws our way and make sure that they become just part of our story, and not the entire book. It takes guts to be willing to learn, to ask for help when we need it, to confront our challenges head on. We just need to accept that, as the saying goes, "we are only as sick as our secrets."

Addiction and the Power of Connection
WITH GENEVIÈVE LAFRENIÈRE

In any discussion of negative thought patterns and behaviours, we must touch on addiction. In Canada, an estimated 6 million people will experience a substance use disorder or addiction at some point in our lives. In the United States, with its larger population, that figure sits at 46.3 million people.

Sober for more than fifteen years, Geneviève Lafrenière is an addiction counsellor and meditation teacher who has been practising in Montreal since 2010. I asked her why so many of us suffer from addiction and how important connection is through the healing process. Here's her insight:

Geneviève Lafrenière: Many of us are addicted to satisfying our deep lack of connection. We haven't learned how to suffer, and/or manage the disconnection from our needs. When someone is compulsive or develops an addiction—social media, alcohol, gambling, drugs, work, food—we look at the purpose this behaviour fulfills—calming, a sense of control, increasing pleasure, vitality, opening up—and we use this to help the person develop skills naturally and potentially achieve abstinence, moderation, and/or healthy living.

Polyvagal theory shows us how to use our nervous system as a personal surveillance system to check whether we are safe and connected—with ourselves, the environment, and others. Why do we have Alcoholics Anonymous and all the other fraternities—Overeaters Anonymous, Gamblers Anonymous, Al-Anon, etc.? Because the strength of the group can provide the safety and communion needed to heal and grow.

The Challenge to Change

In building programs for underserved youth, Jewel collaborates with a team of experts. One of them is psychiatrist, neuroscientist, and bestselling author Dr. Judson Brewer, a thought leader in the field of "self-mastery" and habit breaking (check out *Unwinding Anxiety* and *The Craving Mind*). When it comes to empowering ourselves to change and leave behind negative thought patterns that don't serve us, Dr. Jud is exactly the right person to talk to.

Sophie Grégoire: Why is being aware of our habits and emotions so important?

Dr. Judson Brewer: Awareness is really at the heart of how we develop our habits, whether they're mental or physical, and it's also at the heart of how we break bad habits and foster good habits or helpful habits. Our brains are designed to be tremendously plastic and aren't averse to change. But when our brains find something that works pretty well and they do it for a long time, our brains are going to say, "Hey, this works. This ain't broke; don't fix it." The awareness is actually key for responsibility and giving us power to change.

SG: So, when the brain is addicted, we need to give it a more positive scenario or experience, so it can say, "Okay, fine, I'll quit smoking. I'll do this instead"?

JB: Yes. So, if a behaviour is something rewarding, we're going to keep doing it. I'm thinking of a patient who started drinking because he was anxious, and the drinking would help him numb himself and distract himself from the anxiety. Yet that was starting to cause problems for him. So I had him pay attention to his drinking. It's hard to pay attention when you're intoxicated, so I would have him pay attention afterwards to see what the results were from the drinking, and he was seeing that it really wasn't helping him. It was affecting his health, mentally and physically, and it wasn't helping the anxiety.

There are a couple of ways to help foster stepping out of these habit loops, including finding things that are motivating and rewarding. I call it the "bigger, better offer"—the BBO. For example, we did this study with smoking. We got five times better quit rates than gold-standard treatment by having people pay attention as they smoked their cigarettes. We got a 67 percent reduction in anxiety in people with generalized anxiety disorder, and that was just using a mindfulness app (Unwinding Anxiety). So, in all of the situations that we've looked at, we have found that awareness really can help. One of my favourite internally rewarding behaviours is getting curious.

SG: How does that work?

JB: There are two types of curiosity. One's called "deprivation curiosity," when we're deprived of some information and that drives this itchy, restless urge to go get it. That's not the type of curiosity I'm talking about. If our ancient ancestors heard some rustling in the bushes, deprivation curiosity would get them to go look to see if that's just their sibling or a sabre-toothed tiger waiting to eat them, right?

The type of curiosity that I think of as a superpower is called "interest curiosity." This is when we're truly interested in something and there's no destination in mind; we're just truly interested in that process of discovery that I think of, at the far end, as awe. That's the curiosity that is really helpful. If we're really curious about what somebody thinks about a political issue, about an environmental issue, about a social issue or about the world, we're going to create a connection. Also, if we're truly curious about our own minds, we can learn how our minds work and learn to step out of our old habits. So, for example, one thing I do with my patients, when they have a craving for cigarettes or food or whatever, is have them get really curious about what that craving feels like in their body.

SG: That's torture [laughs].

JB: It might seem like torture at first, but does a craving feel better or does curiosity feel better?

SG: Would you say that mindfulness is a form of playful curiosity?

JB: I would say that playful curiosity, that attitude of curiosity, is at the heart of mindfulness.

SG: Okay, so if we become aware of our own negative habits, are we breaking the cycle of our negative thinking? Are they even related?

JB: Well, negative thinking can become a habit, and there's a lot of research to back that up. There are two main flavours that I deal with as a psychiatrist. One is rumination with depression. So, if somebody is constantly feeling bad and thinking that they're a bad person or regretting things that they've done in life or whatever, this negative rumination about "Oh no, this is bad. It's never going to change" is a habit. That tends to be about the past. The other is the worry thinking that happens with anxiety. There, we can see our minds get stuck in the future, perseverating, worrying. And those are just two examples of pretty strong habit loops that are all about mental behaviours, which is thinking.

SG: When we're stuck in a bad habit, which usually is accompanied by a negative thinking pattern, we're in a fixed mindset. How important is it to be psychologically flexible to gain more perspective on our emotional posture?

JB: A fixed mindset is when we're stuck in a habit and it literally feels closed down. So, if somebody is addicted to something, for example, they're going to feel that drive, that fix: "I have to do this." They're not actually open to change in those moments. So fixed mindset is really about habitual behaviours. Growth mindset is really about this interest curiosity.

SG: When you talk about an awareness of our behaviours, isn't that the core for justice, evolution, and peace, in so many ways?

JB: Yes, it certainly is the core, whether on a personal level if we're trying to change behaviours, or if we're trying to change as a society, or a world level, if we're trying to make our planet a better place.

SG: Can being aware of our emotions and letting go of our fixed mindset be a motivator to learn from our suffering?

JB: That's a great question. I think we naturally let go, like you're talking about, when we're in a safe place and when we're in our growth zone, for example. And then we can explore what it feels like when we're tightly trying to hold on to something, trying to force something, versus just being with whatever's happening and not resisting. So I think of resistance as the opposite of letting go. When we're resisting what's happening, we can just explore that and ask ourselves, "What do I get from resisting what's going to happen anyway?" and then, "What's it like when I allow it to happen?" And that's where the letting go comes in, and we get to discover for ourselves how much better it feels to let go than to hold on.

The reality is that we all tend to hold on to what we are used to. Think about a habit, a relationship, a job, even a favourite pair of shoes. Sometimes we fear that if we step out of our comfort zone, we won't find that same comfort anywhere else. Or maybe we're worried that we'll somehow fail, feel alone, or feel uncertain if we change. But the truth is that we can grow in positive ways when we embrace change, and especially when we let go of things that are holding us back. We can step into the best version of ourselves.

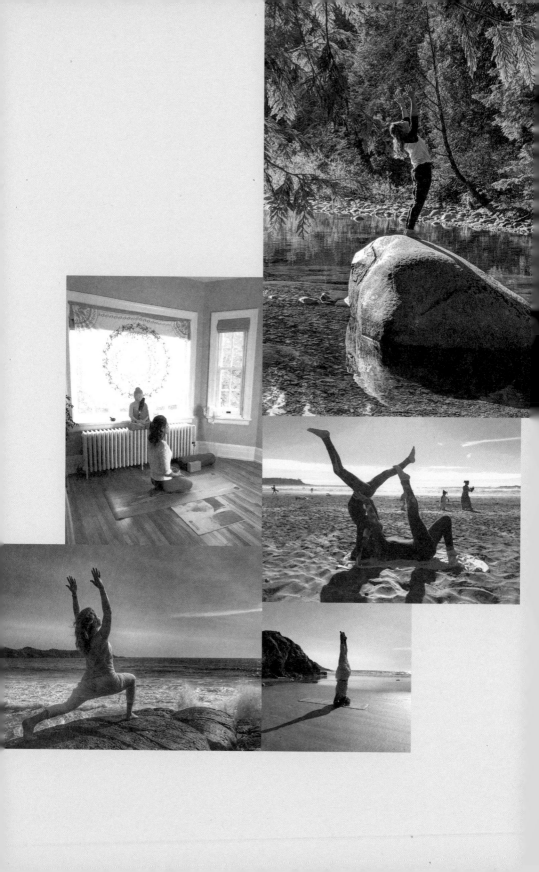

The Gentleness of Here and Now

Mindfulness, Yogic Principles, and the Nerve that Knows Everything

The most fundamental aggression to ourselves, the most fundamental harm we can do to ourselves, is to remain ignorant by not having the courage and the respect to look at ourselves honestly and gently.

PEMA CHÖDRÖN

It's summer, and we are visiting a friend's house. I woke up early, so I perched myself on a barstool to get some writing done in the morning quiet. I'm staring up at some really good bottles of tequila (way too early for that!) when one of my hosts joins me. He's a forty-year-old father who is in good physical shape, has two kids and a wife whom he loves, and a job that makes him happy. He tells me how his ten-year-old daughter asked him to try meditation with her, to help with her anger issues. "I'm not a spiritual dude, you know," he says, "but this stuff kind of seems to work. We sit cross-legged together early in the morning, or before bed once in a while, and we'll put on an app and meditate for ten or fifteen minutes. I used to train a lot at the gym, and I'd sometimes get quite sore. But since I've been meditating, I feel like my body is less sore, and my mind, too. I can't explain it, but it's real."

When I heard him say that, I wanted to jump with joy, and maybe even weep a little! Like my friend, fathers around the world can be a force for change. Within their own families and beyond (as teachers, coaches, and mentors), they can recognize that mental health is as important as physical health, and they can carve out time and space to "walk the walk" by embracing the practices that contribute to well-being. Wouldn't that be an incredible shift in awareness?

Speaking of awareness shifts, I watched a documentary recently called *Stutz*. It's so completely different from anything else I've seen. It could totally change your view of traditional talk therapy. In it, actor and filmmaker Jonah Hill lets us in on the dynamics between him and his thoughtful therapist, Phil Stutz (psychiatrist, author, and creator of The Tools). The two men form a deep bond of trust as they expose their vulnerabilities. Stutz reminds us that there are three realities we can't avoid: pain, uncertainty, and constant work. And if we become more aware of why we feel the way we do, we can come closer to our life force. (In yoga, we call it *prana*; in qigong, they call it *qi*). Stutz says it's the only thing we can work on, and the only force guiding us when we feel lost.

He goes on to explain that the relationship we build with our physical body through nutrition, exercise, and sleep counts for 85 percent of that life force, and that if we work on this, everything else will fall into place. He believes we must be able to create something new in the face of adversity, and that the greater the adversity, the greater the opportunity. But first, we must let go of the guilt we carry, understand the shadowy parts of ourselves, and show true confidence with living in uncertainty. We must develop that faith in our life force and accept the consequences. This process is where true happiness, confidence, and discovery lie.

What I've integrated through my own life experiences and practice is that the true teacher is within us—like with the ten-year-old who told her father that she wanted to try meditation to deal with anger issues, and the father who trusted her and followed her lead. It begins with us. We just need to connect—through courage, presence, and mindfulness—with what we already know.

The Art of Being Present

These days, the word *mindfulness* crops up in all sorts of places—magazine articles, social media feeds, conversations with friends. But what is *mindfulness*, anyway? In the simplest possible terms, it's being aware of and choosing to pay attention to the present moment.

Sounds simple, right? Except for one little thing: we're constantly obsessed with the future. Consider the things that are running through your own mind right now. Are you planning a special outing for next weekend, or a play date for your child? Are you thinking about items you need to add to your (ever-growing) to-do list, or anticipating your next paycheque and figuring out how to juggle the monthly bills? Maybe you're waiting on good news, or worrying that it might be bad. Whatever the case may be, you are not the only one entertaining thoughts like these. So many of us are perpetually projecting ourselves into the future and trying to control what's to come.

The Buddha said, "The past is already gone; the future is not here yet. There's only one moment for you to live, and that is the present moment." Mindfulness is the act of bringing your attention to your own experience and consciously choosing to have positive thoughts and feelings about that experience. When you're mindful, you leave the past behind and you let go of any expectations about the future. That's a tough one, isn't it?

But maybe you've had a sense of that feeling now and again. Have you ever had a moment where you felt particularly in tune with the world and people around you? Perhaps it was while you were sitting on a park bench, or just while staring out a window? It's happened to me. I'll be talking with someone, and while I'm listening intently to their words, I can also sense the underlying emotions. And in that moment, I realize that I truly accept everything about them and about me. That's mindfulness, and the trick to mastering it is to train our bodies and brains to recognize it, to learn how to return to it, and to be able to stay in those moments for longer. When we're able to choose peace and deep presence above everything else, the results are life-changing—both in the moment and sometimes for hours and days to come.

It's good to know, as well, that you can start small. I began with five minutes as soon as I woke up and five minutes before I went to bed each day. Baby steps, but the "slow and steady" approach allowed me to build my mindfulness practice into a habit, just like brushing my teeth. In fact, I felt the results of that mindfulness practice *while* I was brushing my teeth. Instead of thinking about the stressful news of the day, how to save the planet, or the kids' next doctors' appointments, I found myself noticing how the toothbrush massaged my gums, how the water was soothing on my tongue, etc. This same sense of deep presence can be applied to so many of the small tasks you do every single day, with amazing benefits.

All you need to do is show up. And practise, practise, practise.

"Mindfulness allows us to access the being mode and spend time there," says Dr. Zindel Segal. The author of more than ten books, including *The Mindful Way Through Depression* and *The Mindful Way Workbook*, Zindel is also a professor of psychology at the University of Toronto Scarborough, an award-winning clinical psychologist, and an advocate for the relevance of mindfulness-based clinical care in psychiatry and mental health. We spoke about mindfulness and meditation, and how beneficial the practices can be to our mental health and well-being.

> **Sophie Grégoire:** What's your first message for someone who has never meditated, who doesn't even know what mindfulness is?

Dr. Zindel Segal: Don't get caught up in the labels and don't get caught up with huge expectations. When you want to understand what mindfulness is, think about it as a way of paying attention—which is a capacity we already have. In mindfulness practice, what you're trying to do is to develop an acquaintanceship with and befriend emotions. In a sense, you are letting them in so you can investigate them with curiosity and kindness. Eventually, you need to do something about emotions that are difficult. But with mindfulness, the first step really is investigating what is coming up in the body through sensations and not very quickly pushing it away because it feels unpleasant or too hurtful. You don't have to be overwhelmed by emotion; mindfulness is a way of buying yourself a little bit of time to acknowledge and label what's present for you and then decide what you want to do about it. Usually, people rush to get rid of it or deal with it or regulate it.

SG: What's the greatest lesson you've learned through your work with mindfulness?

ZS: People ask me, "Since you've been practising mindfulness all this time, have you really changed as a person?" And I would say no, I haven't really changed dramatically, but I would say that there are some things I find harder to do. I find it harder to gossip and judge other people. It doesn't mean I'm perfect [laughs], but I notice it. And I also find myself a little bit more willing to help other people. I do feel like I have this thing underneath me that I can always turn to that gives me perspective when other stuff is coming at me. And I think that's really valuable.

SG: Can we talk about the difference between meditation and mindfulness?

ZS: Meditation is the way you develop mindfulness. Mindfulness is an awareness that allows you to be in the present moment and not judge what you find. When you slow down and eat mindfully, you're more aware of the food you're eating, you're

233

more aware of how it tastes, you're more aware of the muscles in your mouth, etc.

SG: In a society where the drugs of choice are intensity and distraction, how can mindfulness help us better understand our own addictions?

ZS: Well, I think mindfulness is the antidote to distraction and intensity, because what mindfulness suggests is that the richness found in a moment of being present can easily compete with the richness found in intensity and continuous attention to whatever external factors are demanding that we are present for them. And you can only do that if you're able to let go. Mindfulness is very much a training of letting go.

SG: What do you mean by "letting go"? Letting go of what?

ZS: That's a good question, because I think sometimes it can be misinterpreted. If only you could let go of your anger or your blame, you'd be fine. I'm not talking about that general "letting go." When you practise mindfulness, you can see that the mind wants to have certain goals and objectives. It's letting go of the mind needing to create an experience for you before you actually have that experience, and letting things come to you in a way where you might be surprised, but you're still staying with the experience because you're curious about it.

SG: Our lives these days are so fast-paced. People are drained physically and emotionally. Can mindfulness help restore the brain, and therefore have calming effects on our lives?

ZS: The practice of meditation involves a calming of the nervous system—just closing your eyes and sitting and doing nothing in one place can cause the nervous system to settle and not be actively engaged in goal-directed behaviour. So there is a natural calming. And then, once you are able to achieve that pretty regularly, that's an additional way you're restoring the brain. It's just a way of being with your experience that involves investigation, attending, curiosity, and kindness. I think those qualities are very restorative, because there's usually an imbalance between how much time we spend in the doing mode and how much time we spend in the being mode. Our attention gets hijacked by all of these external cues that tell us, "You've got to be on Twitter; you've got to be on Insta; you've got to be on TikTok; you've got to be watching this show; you've got to buy this." That's the attention economy. And some people think there's nowhere else to pay attention. But what mindfulness and meditation are telling us is that, actually, there is this other place to pay attention from.

SG: By being mindful, are we becoming more maternal/paternal to and with ourselves? Can we learn, through mindfulness, that care we might not have been given as children?

ZS: I think that is very accurate. When you're able to honour your own experience by paying attention to it, there is an inherent kindness that you are engaging in. You're saying you're good enough to be attended to, you're good enough to understand and investigate what's going on for you.

In the years that have passed since I first began a mindfulness practice—with those five-minute sessions—it has become an important part of my life. I depend on it to clear my mind at the beginning of the day, so I can start fresh, and to do the same at the end of the day, so I go to bed without a million thoughts racing through my brain. But when it comes to doing the work of "investigating what's going on for me," as Zindel put it, there is also another practice that has become just as vital to my well-being.

The Wisdom of Yoga

Sometimes I like to look back through the diary I kept while studying to become a yoga teacher. Recently, I came across my own words: "Go where life unfolds: within. When you avoid silence, you avoid yourself. Befriend silence and you will befriend yourself." I should maybe stick that on my fridge door!

Yoga has helped me to reconnect with myself in deeply meaningful ways. Simply put, it allows us to keep a cool head on a warm body—meaning you can push your physical boundaries while keeping a sense of equanimity in your mind.

It is a reminder of an undeniable duality: I am only a particle of dust *and* I am a sacred part of the universe. I practise yoga and meditation to declutter my mind; they make everything feel less complicated and confusing. No one has described it better than master teacher and guru B. K. S. Iyengar. In *Light on Yoga*, he wrote, "It is the supreme goal of yoga, the greatest result of meditation, to become so empty and clear, like an open window, that the light of the sun and the breath of the wind can move freely through you, thereby transcending the limitations of the human ego with all its petty concerns. It is total surrender. It is total understanding. It is total compassion."

I'll admit it: when I was a teenager, I thought only hippies and monks practised meditation and yoga. I had no clue, really, what they were. It wasn't until I was about thirty that I learned more. Justin and I had bought a condo on Dollard Street in Montreal from a well-respected and kind yoga teacher. I'd recently grown more curious about the practice, so I thought I'd try a class at her nearby studio. What an experience! It was physically demanding, and the movements were interesting. The teacher set a good pace, and her comments kept me intrigued. Most of all, though, I was shocked by the emotion I felt during class. I felt like I was properly guided to use my body strength, my patience, my mental and physical flexibility (trust me, I couldn't do all the poses at first), and my openness to try something new without judging myself. I felt welcomed.

In a matter of an hour, it felt like I had found another home. When we were asked to come into corpse pose at the end (a lying-down pose called *savasana* in Sanskrit), I felt a huge release. Tears were rolling softly, so softly. I was smiling. I had no idea how to explain it, but I knew I wanted more. It was as if yoga had been patiently waiting for me to find its wisdom.

I soon came to understand that yoga is simply a practice where you can show up for yourself, often in the company of other peaceful humans who are interested in diving deeper into the body and the soul. I learned that the physical practice of yoga has been used for centuries as a way to prepare the body for meditation. It clears the mind of debris so we are ready for greater self-compassion, wisdom, non-attachment, and acceptance of all life's imperfections, including our own. A calm mind and body amid the noise and the chaos of life is a necessity, not a luxury.

I began with hatha yoga (*hatha* means "force," or "to persist in something with effort"), which wasn't too difficult for me to learn, and I enjoyed the three fundamental elements: poses (moving asanas), breathing techniques (pranayama), and meditation (dhyana). But as I advanced, I had to develop patience for new poses that didn't come so easily. I never thought I would be able to do the splits in my late forties, but it happened as I continued to dedicate myself to practice. Yoga became a tool to keep my mind at peace and my body in balance, and it brought me so much joy that I wanted others to feel as grounded and happy as I was. By the time I was in my early thirties, I'd completed my two-hundred-hour teacher training.

I could have learned and practised all day long. From the history of yoga to anatomy to tantric philosophy, everything was fascinating. I practised with discipline and started a half-hour meditation ritual during early mornings. Meditating didn't come easily at first, and I would wiggle a lot as my legs would occasionally go numb (they still do!). But my love of silence allowed me to be patient, and I came to understand that meditating wasn't something I needed to be "good" at; the simple act of sitting in silence was what calmed the body and mind. When I let go of my desire to "perform" at meditation, something switched inside me. I learned once that meditating is like meeting your inner lover. That really resonated. Ask yourself: Can you be patient, caring, loving, attentive, truly intimate, and gentle with yourself? For me, it is a rebellious act of pure love and deep listening. But trust me when I tell you that I still don't have it all together, and I'm continuously trying to do my best all while stumbling and making mistakes in my own life.

Once my teacher training was complete, I was permitted to lead a few free community classes at the studio. I totally overprepared, but some of my friends and family showed up and offered great support. I kept up with the instructing for the next few months, until we moved to Ottawa in 2013. I was soon busy with all of the usual stuff that comes with relocating, from school registrations and finding a doctor and a dentist to signing the kids up for community classes to getting to know my new surroundings. I still made time to practise, though, right until the last days of my pregnancy with Hadrien (he wasn't born a yogi, but he *was* a very mellow baby). I picked it up again a couple of months after giving birth. All three of our kids have seen my yoga practice evolve through the years, and have even joined me now and again. But you know how it is: anything their (very cool) mom does isn't cool, right? Still, I see how easily they fall asleep after I have guided them through a yoga nidra session and adjusted their bodies into relaxation. (*Yoga nidra* or "yogic sleep" is a state of consciousness between waking and sleeping. While we remain still, we observe and scan different parts of the body, guided by the cues of a teacher. Yoga nidra diminishes symptoms of anxiety by bringing the body and mind into a state of calm. It can be practised any time during the day or before sleep.) I hope they carry that memory and its lessons with them into adulthood.

I also expanded my practice when opportunities arose. One year, I accompanied a close friend to the Omega Institute for Holistic Studies in Rhinebeck, New York, where I attended my first-ever Afro Flow yoga class. Afro Flow yoga is the connection of yogic principles, spirituality, dances of the African diaspora, and the intrinsic expression of movement through nature's elements. It was a unique and enriching experience.

Sometimes you go to yoga, and sometimes yoga comes to you—even in the unlikeliest of places.

Hadrien had always been reluctant to try camp (do you think that might have had something to do with his big brother mentioning that he didn't like it?), so when a mom at his school suggested we take part in a short parent-and-child stay at a camp near Mont-Tremblant, I signed us up. I figured sharing a tent under the stars and meeting up with his friend's family might be just the thing to show Hadrien how magical camping can be. When we arrived, sleeping bags and pillows in tow, I made my way to the little reception office to register. The camp director came over to say hello, and reminded me that we'd completed our yoga instructor training together in Montreal. What a small world.

The first two days were a predictable mix of good and not-so-good. We decorated our tent with little battery-operated lights and read stories at night, and Hadrien headed off to the cafeteria in the morning and drank Kool-Aid for breakfast, which stained his tongue purple. That was all great. But we also tried mountain biking (Didi scraped his knees bloody in the first five minutes) and played in the water (he was shivering, with lips turning blue, after fifteen minutes). I wanted to go canoeing and paddleboarding (he didn't). His shoes and many of our clothes were wet from the rain and just wouldn't dry. We were sleep-deprived, *and* he refused to shower. He did find solace in woodworking, though, and carved a beautiful little wooden paddle for his dad.

Sometime during that second day, I realized I was craving a little solace of my own. I hadn't practised yoga since we'd arrived, so I talked to a couple of the parents and the camp director about teaching a class. We found a space near a fireplace in the counsellors' cabin, big enough to fit the twelve or so people who showed up. It felt like everyone in the room needed a breather as much as I did.

I began by having everyone stand up and let go of their expectations for that class or themselves. The room went completely silent. We started out slowly and then gradually moved more rapidly to raise our heartbeats and stretch our bodies. When I heard deep breaths and saw sweaty faces, I knew we were all working hard, and I reminded everyone to relax their foreheads and throats. Then, gradually, I slowed the cadence again, allowing our heart rates to slow as well. We moved on to stretches and then savasana.

Observing the group with their outstretched arms resembling wings, I thought we all looked a bit like angels. It was time for yoga nidra. With a low voice, I guided the class through this observation of the motionless body. I lowered my voice even more and guided everyone into deep relaxation. Some fell asleep, some had an emotional release and sobbed, and all experienced a profound release— completely normal responses. I saw these people, most of whom I'd never met before, completely at peace. For a little while, at least, they'd left their daily troubles behind and found a state of bliss. I was so happy to see the look of beatitude on their faces.

It's always been my experience that the practice of yoga and the letting go it allows make room for deep and meaningful conversations. Two of the students, in their twenties, sought me out afterwards. One, a young woman, told me that she'd been on sleeping pills for most of her life and suffered from crippling anxiety. A natural athlete, she was looking for ways to take control of her life and lower her stress levels. Her boyfriend, a long-time competitive swimmer, learned at sixteen that he had a congenital heart disease. He underwent a serious operation, was bedridden for a long time, and had doctors tell him he would never train again. He defied the odds and now competed in triathlons, but admitted that performance anxiety was making him unhappy. He wondered how he might rebalance his life.

Every time someone shares a story like this with me after a class, I am reminded of two things: first, how much weight we all carry on our shoulders, and second, how connected we are in our quest for well-being. Our problems may be different, but they can leave us wondering the same things: How will we make it to the next moment, or the next day? How can we repair this relationship? How can we be a better spouse, parent, friend, employee? Learning how to feel our way through the fog of life demands that we get in touch with and trust our inner compass. To me, yoga is an invitation to be open and honest

240

Performance Anxiety

In chapter 4, we heard from Olympian Mark Tewksbury on the importance of living an authentic life. But like the young man who spoke with me after the yoga class at camp, Mark has experienced performance anxiety. In fact, it nearly derailed his swimming career. Thanks to an insightful coach and his own perseverance, he was able to change his mindset and continue to thrive.

Sophie Grégoire: Tell me more about your experience with performance anxiety.

Mark Tewksbury: During the last year of my Olympic career, a new coach noticed that I had changed the way I spoke of my own performance. I kept talking about how amazing my competition looked and how nothing we were doing was working. Without even knowing it, my negative, limited thinking was literally holding me back.

SG: What does this negative thinking sound like?

MT: There I was, second-best in the world, and the core of it was, "You can't beat this guy; you're never going to be good enough to win the Olympics." You don't have to be an Olympian to be thinking that way. Feeling overwhelmed by life, nervous about a new job, scared to death because you're about to have your first baby—it's all about letting go of what you can't control. Writing down the negative stuff was liberating, as it left space for what we *could* do something about. It took some time to change the way I showed up in the world. But it came.

with yourself and others. It creates moments where we can come closer and share the collective story of our well-being.

I'm not suggesting that yoga is the solution to every mental health issue. But it is an accessible, affordable, secular, efficient, authentic, compassionate, and lifelong practice. And there is no doubt that it can improve our lives. Dr. Amy Wheeler, co-founder of Optimal State Yoga Therapy, has seen the positive impact of the practice on herself and the hundreds of students she has taught through the years. Amy's purpose in life has been to educate people about yoga, psychology, and wellness. She's been part of a team that has developed numerous yoga therapy research projects, including working with researchers at Vanderbilt University on metabolic syndrome, colon and rectal cancer, ovarian and uterine cancer, and low-back surgery. We spoke about yoga's many benefits for mind, body, and spirit.

> **Sophie Grégoire:** Amy, what's the scientific evidence that supports yoga's benefits for psychological and physical health?
>
> **Dr. Amy Wheeler:** The research that's coming out about yoga and yoga therapy is so phenomenal, especially with how it inter- sects with mental health and neurophysiology. We're really starting to understand that the neural pathways in our brain and through our nervous system into our body are heavily impacted by movement, breath, and mental focus. Last year, I was diagnosed with cancer. The ability of yoga to help me through my cancer surgery was shocking to me. Yoga has also taught me humility—that I don't know what I think I know, and that there are a lot of gaps in my perception. It's taught me to be kind and have empathy.
>
> **SG:** Can we talk about the main impacts yoga has on the brain?
>
> **AW:** Yoga helps with our executive functioning and planning, which is located in the prefrontal cortex. It has an impact on our amygdala, which is our fear centre; it tends to lessen our reactivity when we're feeling fearful. I would also say it

affects the corpus callosum, which is like the superhighway between the left and right brain. It's the ability of the right brain and left brain to talk to each other that makes us a happier, healthier human.

SG: How does the practice of yoga affect our nervous system?

AW: Yoga allows my perception to shift when I'm in a state of sympathetic activity in my nervous system—which activates the fight-or-flight response—versus a parasympathetic state, which is responsible for the relax-rest-digest-heal mode. So the same situation could be right here in front of me, but if I'm stressed out, I'm going to perceive it very differently than if I'm feeling relaxed. I would argue that our goal is not just to stay relaxed; our goal is to be rotating the nervous system, where you're able to go up into a stress response and get back down, and go up and get back down. Because inevitably life is going to cause us to go into the stress response, so we can't just be a noodle sitting there [laughs].

SG: And what about digestion—because so many people have digestive issues these days.

AW: I've learned from my teachers in India that digestion is physical, it's mental, emotional, and spiritual. And everything that comes at us all day long is like food. Maybe not physical food, but it's spiritual food or mental and emotional food, and we need to be very careful and protect ourselves from letting too much of the wrong food in. So, just as I'm making healthy choices for my physical digestion, am I also making healthy choices about the mental, emotional, and spiritual stimulus that I'm allowing to come into myself? It's worth looking at digestion as food, but also in a much broader sense of "What do I allow in and what do I say, 'No, thank you,' to?"

SG: What would you like to say to parents or youths who are reluctant when it comes to yoga—especially our boys?

AW: I think young men have this idea about yoga being a class with a bunch of women in yoga tights—and we need to break that stereotype. I work with a lot of young men on their mental and emotional self-awareness. They track their mental and emotional awareness throughout the day on our Optimal State mobile app and then they send their data to me. There comes a point where they can care for themselves: "I'm really out of balance this week, but I know what to do now." They are learning how to make themselves feel better.

SG: Unbelievable. Every youth needs that. Finally, what is *salutogenesis*?

AW: Salutogenesis is a sense of flourishing and well-being and feeling well. It's the opposite of pathogenesis. Yoga can affect this, and it can get us to that state of what they're now calling "thrivancy." It's saying we have to take people beyond resilience. Resilience is like, "Can I hang on for dear life in this crazy world?" Thrivancy is five steps higher than that. I don't just want to survive or be resilient in a dysfunctional system; I want to learn to thrive.

Yoga creates a sense of coming home, which is the most intimate place that you can visit inside of yourself, and in our relationships as well.

SG: Coming home and sitting with our heartbrokenness. Yoga makes me feel safer while I travel in that realm.

AW: If you can feel safe inside yourself even while living with a broken heart, you have lived a state of yoga.

That sense of "coming home" and of feeling safe inside myself is exactly why yoga and mindfulness have become so important to me. Together, these practices allow me to better know my authentic self. They also provide some of the tools I need to help bring my nervous system back into balance when life throws me a curveball or two. But they aren't the only tools at our disposal. Recently, for example, I've learned about a built-in system—or nerve, actually—that can really help us out.

A Simple Practice to Calm Anxiety

WITH NINA ZOLOTOW

Nina Zolotow, author of *Yoga for Times of Change*, knows just how powerful a few simple practices can be. This one takes only three minutes, and you can do it just about anywhere:

1. Go to a nearby table (or desk) and move a chair several inches away from the table. Then sit on the chair, facing the table, with your buttocks near the front of the chair. (If there isn't a table or desk nearby, you can do this standing up by finding a chest of drawers or countertop that is the right height to rest your arms and head on. Walk far enough away from the support so you can bend toward it from your hip joints without overly rounding your spine.)

2. Bend forward from your hip joints—keeping your spine long— and rest your forehead on your folded arms on the desk. Try gently tugging your forehead skin down toward your eyebrows.

3. Once you have settled into a comfortable position, try bringing your attention to your breath. Briefly observe both your inhalations and your exhalations.

4. Now bring your awareness to your next exhalation and notice when you reach the end of it. Without straining, lengthen your exhalation just a bit (about as long as it takes to say the word *peace*). Inhale naturally. Then lengthen your next exhalation in the same way and inhale naturally.

5. Keep practising this way, lengthening your exhalation just a bit and inhaling naturally. If you lose track of what you're doing, it's okay. Just resume with your next exhalation.

6. If focusing on your breath increases your anxiety, try mentally repeating a calming phrase or word to yourself, such as "I can get through this" or even just "Peace."

7. Stay for three or more minutes. When you're ready to finish the exercise, breathe naturally for a few rounds and then slowly lift your head up. When you're ready to stand up, do that slowly, too.

Meet the Vagus Nerve

I've had so many revelations while writing this book, but the biggest one might be that our capacity for compassion emerges from a regulated nervous system.

Yup. You read that right. Scientist and professor Stephen Porges's polyvagal theory explains, in part, how an unregulated nervous system makes it difficult for a person to build a relationship of trust with themselves and with others. Dr. Porges's pioneering studies are based on the neurophysiological foundations of attachment, communication, emotions, and self-regulation, and revelations about the vagus nerve have allowed us to better understand its role and functions in restoring balance to our nervous system. Although some experts say his theory remains unproven, many respected scientists and practitioners have praised his work. Dr. Gabor Maté, for example, describes it as a "brilliant contribution to understanding the nervous system and its functioning." He adds that while it doesn't explain everything, he has studied it in detail and uses it in his own work.

In order to understand polyvagal theory, we need a quick refresher on our nervous system. As we saw in chapter 1, the autonomic (meaning "involuntary") nervous system has two main branches. The sympathetic nervous system is associated with our fight-or-flight response, while the parasympathetic nervous system regulates a relaxation response, sometimes referred to as "rest and digest." Ideally, these two branches are in a state of balance, or homeostasis. When that happens, we are relaxed, open, and calm. Our heart rate and breathing are regular, our digestion is good, and we're able to make authentic and deep connections with those around us. But in our current culture, we are too often out of balance. Maybe we're dealing with an anxiety disorder (as are an estimated 10 percent of adults in Canada and 19 percent of adults in the United States) or maybe we're simply reacting to the ups and downs of everyday life—a breakup, a sick parent, or even being late for a meeting at work. Whatever the cause, stress sends our parasympathetic nervous system into that fight-or-flight response, and if we go there too often, or stay too long, it takes a toll on our bodies. Our heart rate rises, our breathing becomes shallow, and we can

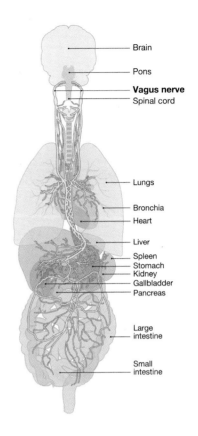

feel afraid, anxious, and even angry. In order to restore our nervous system to a balanced state, we need to trigger a relaxation response and come back to a place of comfort and safety.

This is where the vagus nerve—the main component of the parasympathetic nervous system—makes its grand entrance. *Vagus* is the Latin word for "wandering," which makes it a fitting name for the only cranial nerve that extends beyond the head and neck. It emerges from the top of the brain stem and, after leaving the skull, enters the upper neck area behind each ear. The nerve then travels, splitting into two main branches, through the neck to the throat and vocal cords, and carries on to the heart, lungs, stomach, liver, kidney, spleen, gall bladder, and pancreas. Finally, it extends to the small intestine and part of the large intestine. The dorsal branch regulates the organs below the diaphragm, while the ventral branch is responsible for everything above, including the muscles of the heart, face, and lungs. Simply put, the vagus nerve regulates swallowing, vocalization, breathing, heart rate, blood pressure, digestion, immune response, facial expressions, the microbes found in our intestines, and so much more. If you're not impressed yet, you never will be. The vagus nerve—*your* vagus nerve—is a player when it comes to your mood, how you interact with others, your anxiety level, sleep, digestion, and how well you recover from illness.

It's no surprise, then, that the vagus nerve—which can send signals of relaxation or anger, calm or nervousness to the brain—is critical when it comes to restoring balance in our nervous system and keeping us in a relaxed and open state. This is the knowledge at the heart of Dr. Stephen Porges's polyvagal theory (see the box below for a primer), which explains the interrelationship of the vagus nerve and the autonomic nervous system. Broadly speaking, the vagus nerve is a direct, two-way communication system between brain and body. And, once we know how, we can encourage that communication system to work in our favour by sending the right signals to the brain. Developing a strong "vagal tone" is a key part of that process, and can help us improve our overall health, including our levels of adaptability, emotional flexibility, physical stability, and capacity to respond to trauma. In fact, many practising psychotherapists use polyvagal theory to treat anxiety and post-traumatic stress disorder.

The Polyvagal Theory

Dr. Stephen Porges's polyvagal theory explains how the two branches of the vagus nerve regulate facial expressions, heart rate and breath, and digestion. It helps us understand three neural circuits that support different responses to the world around us, which is why it's been called "the science of connection." The three responses are:

OPENNESS TO SOCIAL ENGAGEMENT—the behaviours we exhibit when we feel safe. This response is regulated by the parasympathetic nervous system, specifically by the *ventral branch* of the vagus nerve. When we are open in this way, our bodies are calm (our heart rate and breathing are regular), and we feel peace, happiness, and curiosity about what is going on around us. This is reflected in our facial expressions, which are natural and relaxed. We can easily listen to and understand others and relate on an emotional level.

FIGHT-OR-FLIGHT RESPONSE—when we are mobilized to respond to a stressor. This response is regulated by the *sympathetic nervous system*. When we are in fight-or-flight mode, we feel anxious or afraid, and our heart rate and breath speed up. Our facial expressions may reflect our fear, or they may be less animated as all of our energy goes into preparing to respond. We may misread signals from those around us, interpreting neutral expressions as aggressive, or fearful expressions as angry. This makes relationships difficult.

SHUT-DOWN RESPONSE—when we are immobilized in response to a stressor. This response is regulated by the *dorsal branch* of the vagus nerve. When we are in shut-down mode, our heart rate and breathing slows. We can feel disassociated or numb, and our expression may appear "spaced out." We may feel hopeless or a sense of shame, and it may be difficult for us to speak. We are not relating to others in this state.

What polyvagal theory makes clear is that the vagus nerve plays a key role in both the social and shut-down responses. By stimulating the vagus nerve in the right ways, we can help our nervous system deal with stressors more efficiently and return us to a balanced, relaxed state.

Learning about the vagus nerve has been such an eye-opener. If we think of it like an antenna or radar, constantly receiving and sending signals to the brain from the body and the environment, we can immediately understand how important relationships and connection are. With the help of this nerve, we actually pick up on the energy of other people's nervous systems and incorporate that into our responses to the world. We function best when the communication between our vagus nerve and the brain is fluid and unobstructed. This allows us to both scan our surroundings for threats or danger *and* have access to a relaxed state of safety.

Acclaimed clinician, speaker, and author Deb Dana (*Anchored: How to Befriend Your Nervous System Using Polyvagal Theory*) is an expert on the vagus nerve and the many ways it can affect our sense of well-being. "Everything that happens to us begins in the body, then gets fed up to the brain, and the brain makes a story about what's happening in our nervous system," she told me, explaining that any symptoms we may feel—from a racing heart to a dry mouth—are the "nervous system trying to tell you something. That's really what it is. And those symptoms are universal, because the nervous system is the common denominator in our human experience." Oh, did I have questions for Deb!

Sophie Grégoire: Can you explain the ventral and dorsal parts of our vagus nerve?

Deb Dana: From the diaphragm upward, we refer to the ventral portion of the vagus nerve, and from the diaphragm down is the dorsal portion. They have different responsibilities, but they're part of the same nerve, so they work together, which is so beautiful.

The ventral portion is that place where we can feel safe in the world, where our system is regulated. This is a place of possibility. The dorsal portion, when it's working on its own, takes us into a survival state—into shutdown, into collapse, into disconnection. But when it's acting in combination with the ventral, it brings us healthy digestion and this beautiful capacity to become still and reflect and take things in.

SG: It sounds almost as if it's our own internal pace- and peacemaker.

DD: It *is* both a pace- and peacemaker. The sympathetic nervous system, when it is working with the ventral portion of the vagus nerve, brings you energy to move through your day. It helps regulate your heart rate and your breath. When it's acting on its own as a survival response, it brings us into a fight-or-flight state.

So our nervous system has this lovely capacity to multi-task. And yet if ventral is not overseeing the system, sympathetic and dorsal can only perform their survival roles.

SG: What relationship would you draw between the childhood attachment bond and how we find ourselves in relationship with our body related to polyvagal theory?

DD: Polyvagal theory would say that your nervous system state is the platform for the attachment style we create. We need our survival strategies; they're important for all of us. We also need to be able to sense safety. And that's challenging for many of us who grew up without that environment of safety as a child. So nervous system comes first. And then out of that, we build patterns in our relationships. Compassion emerges from a regulated nervous system.

If we are in a survival state—either fight or flight, or collapse-shutdown—we cannot access compassion. Not because we don't want to, but because we're unable to. So compassion, self-compassion, curiosity, even—we have to have enough ventral in our system, active and alive, so that we can access those lovely places of feeling.

SG: How do we befriend our nervous system?

DD: Well, the first thing we need to do is turn toward it. We need to bring into explicit awareness everything that's happening below the level of our consciousness. We need to bring attention to the levels of regulation and dysregulation so that we can become active operators of our nervous system. We can find ways to anchor more in ventral and find ways to return from sympathetic and dorsal, which we go into many times a day.

That's the normal human experience. It's not that we are always in a regulated state; that's not achievable or even desirable. But when we befriend our nervous system, we can notice what's going on, name it, bring it into awareness, and then turn toward it. The easiest way is to just listen for a moment, because if you listen in, that autonomic nervous system will speak to you.

SG: So polyvagal theory and techniques can be used, in part, to heal from post-traumatic stress, eating disorders, anxiety, depression?

DD: Anxiety is a symptom of a nervous system that can't find regulation and is stuck in sympathetic, mobilizing, anxious energy. Depression might be thought of as a nervous system that's stuck in disconnection and despair. Your biology is trying to give you a message. If we can listen and tune in and find more moments of regulation, those symptoms begin to change, they reduce, they even resolve sometimes.

SG: We're all one trauma away from one another. It feels somehow as if the planet has a central nervous system and we're all little nervous systems connected to it.

DD: I love that. I say we are inextricably connected to nervous systems around the globe—every nervous system. As I move through the world, I am sending messages to every being around me. Whether I'm personally connecting with those people or not doesn't matter. My nervous system is either sending a welcome, because I'm regulated, or a warning, because I'm dysregulated. And then other nervous systems pick up on that. And then we begin to see these large groups of people who are dysregulated in sympathetic fight or flight, or dysregulated in dorsal hopelessness and despair.

What I have been teaching recently, or preaching is probably more like it, is that unless we are anchored in ventral, change cannot happen. Biologically, our system is closed to change unless we are regulated. And so we need to have a tipping point of people who are anchored in ventral so that we can begin to have the difficult conversations that need to happen for us to come together as humans. I can't do that if I'm in survival mode.

SG: Okay, so if we want to change our story, we must first change our state. What do you hope people will say about how we treated ourselves in ten, twenty, fifty, one hundred years?

DD: My hope is that as my grandchildren become adults, conversations like this one will be common in families. That's really how I think change will happen.

Are you ready to befriend your own nervous system? Next time you feel your heart beat faster, or you feel weak and anxious, or you feel stuck in lethargy, make sure to listen to the messages your body is sending. You can then take easy steps that will help you return to a calm and safe state. In the next chapter, we'll explore how creativity, humour, and a little good mischief all have a central role to play in keeping ourselves healthy—and happy!

Two Simple Exercises for Vagus Nerve Stimulation

I'm sure we'd all like to access a ventral state of calmness and safety, right? Here are two quick and easy exercises we can do anytime and almost anywhere.

EXERCISE #1: FOCUSED GAZE

Lie on the floor or on a bed. You may bend your knees, placing your feet flat on the surface, or have your legs stretched out with a pillow under the knees if needed. Breathe in deeply through your nose and then exhale deeply, sighing the breath out through your mouth. Now clasp your hands and place them behind your head at the lowest part of your skull, with your elbows pointing out to the sides. In this position, your pinkies should be close to the base of your skull and your thumbs naturally facing downward on your neck. Keep breathing deeply and turn your head to the right as far as possible. Then do the same to the left. Repeat a couple of times on each side. When you're done, bring your head back to centre, with your eyes looking to the ceiling. Without moving your head, bring only your gaze (both eyes) to the right and find a point to focus on. This may feel odd at first, but your eyes will adjust. Keep your gaze focused to the right, without moving your head, for a count of thirty seconds to one minute. You may notice that your mouth is watering, or other sensations may be felt in your face or in your belly. Once the time is up, bring your gaze back to the ceiling and relax. Now repeat the process on your left side. Finally, bring your gaze back to the ceiling and take one last deep breath in and out. Try to slow down your movements and steps for a couple of minutes after this practice; this way, you'll avoid stressing your newly relaxed system.

EXERCISE #2: SAVOURING

Deb Dana's practice of savouring is about seeing and celebrating the little things in everyday life. We savour when we recognize an experience in the moment, when we remember a moment and reminisce, and when we anticipate an upcoming experience. When we bring these moments into awareness and spend just a short amount of time actively engaged in attending to them, the benefits are both immediate, as we feel anchored in ventral safety, and longer term, with gains in physical and emotional well-being.

Savouring is a brief three-step, twenty-to-thirty-second practice that easily fits into the flow of a day.

1. First, attend. Bring a ventral vagal moment (a moment where you felt safe and social, calm, curious, joyful) into awareness and stop to notice it.
2. Next, appreciate the moment. Stay with your awareness.
3. Finally, amplify. Hold the moment in focused awareness for twenty to thirty seconds. Feel the fullness of the moment.

You may find it easy to savour your experience for twenty seconds, and in that case, you could extend your appreciation to thirty seconds. Some may feel it's dangerous to feel so good, and that something bad might happen. This is not an uncommon experience. When this happens, start slowly with five or ten seconds and build toward twenty or thirty. Find the amount of time that supports your ability to attend, appreciate, and amplify. Over time, you'll find your capacity to savour will increase.

For more exercises from Deb Dana, check out her book *Polyvagal Exercises for Safety and Connection: 50 Client-Centered Practices.*

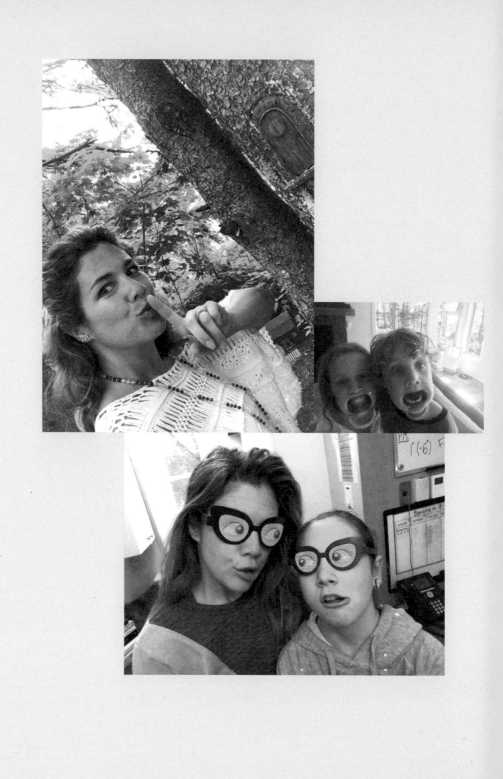

10

Time for Play!

Humour, Fun, and Creativity for the Mind and Soul

Childhood dreams are forever stuffed in our souls.

Take them out and play sometimes.

ANGIE WEILAND-CROSBY

If there's one thing I've learned in life, it's that you have to be open to moments of playfulness and humour when they present themselves. As a mom, I try to give my children the space they need to fully express and feel their emotions, so we can discuss their roots and gain some perspective. One night, when we were cuddled up under the covers after story time, Hadrien, who was eight at the time, told me he couldn't fall asleep. "There are too many thoughts in my head and I can't just stop them," he said.

"Oh, my love, I understand," I answered. "Here's a little trick: pretend there's a tiny little door somewhere at the top of your brain. Now open that door and let all the thoughts, emotions, and ideas be free; let them drift softly out into the air for the night . . . Your mind is now empty, spacious, and calm."

Silence.

Then Hadrien looked at me and said, "Hmm. Yes. Wow. Now I understand why you keep forgetting everything, Mom."

After we got over our giggle fit, Hadrien's mind was calmer, and he was able to drift off to sleep. And I was left thinking about how laughter really is the cure for so many ills.

I love to laugh, and to make others laugh, too. To me, laughter and playfulness are a natural form of reverence for life, and a healing tool for the mind and the soul. They allow us to shoulder our troubles together so they feel lighter, almost weightless. Some even say that the sacred can't come in if we haven't laughed! Oh . . . do I love that one.

As far back as I can remember, I've had a flame of mischief in me. Whether jumping over fences, mud puddles, or society's rules, I craved a slight sense of disobedience, though it was never malicious. I'd climb trees a tad too high, and secretly spy on my best friend's brothers or a camp counsellor changing her clothes (I know, bad!). The desire to play practical jokes on friends or co-opt them into a bit of mischief has always been in me. I come by it naturally: my dad and his brother constantly played tricks or performed stunts just to get belly laughs. When my father was a kid, he would walk up to an auntie or family friend with a box of chocolates and encourage them to open it and pick one. But instead of holding tasty treats, the box was filled with garter snakes! His sense of humour was contagious, and it helped me lower the "drama meter" on some difficult moments in my life.

My mom's brothers (the coolest uncles) were also quite the pranksters. It definitely runs in the family—although it seemed like that mischievousness was traditionally associated with masculine energy. Well, I totally balanced that out. Laughter was like a therapy to me. I bet you've felt the same way at some point in your life. It's not surprising. Many experts agree that play, humour, curiosity, and the ability to not take ourselves too seriously have important benefits to our brains, and therefore our well-being. With that in mind, this chapter is dedicated to many forms of fun, starting with play.

The Power of Play

Do you remember the games you played when you were young? The endless hours of hide-and-seek, the intricate "let's pretend" scenarios where you and a friend would create an entire make-believe world? Good times. As adults, many of us have, sadly, left those days behind. But we—and our brains—need the space of play to calm down and reset. Gordon Neufeld told me that playfulness is so good for the brain that it serves an equivalent function to rest; he called it "active rest." "Play allows for maximum neural plasticity and maximum restoration, without having to be asleep," he said. The instinct to play sits right alongside the instinct to breathe, and the simple act of playing can make us feel safe even when we are not."

Gordon has seen this at work in Ukraine, during the war with Russia. "I have had a number of addresses with Ukrainian teachers during this war. And Ukrainian mothers, or those who are working with Ukrainian mothers in Poland. And the message was simple: when bombs are falling down and a child is at play, they feel safe even though they're not. Which is what the brain needs for restoration."

Dr. Allan Schore also had some wonderful insight: "Play is really the great source of positive emotions and the ability to have joy in one's life. And the ability to feel is key there. But it's one thing to play by myself, and it's an entirely different thing to play with another human being. When two people play with each other, they're synchronizing, nervous system to nervous system. And play also allows us to cope with the novel, the new, not just the familiar."

I can attest to that. Humour and play have allowed me to set a positive and open tone in my life, and to adapt to different situations with a certain sense of perspective. I pinned electrodes on the back of the science teacher's lab coat while he was walking around the class. I hung our adored geography teacher's keys from the dangling cord of the projector screen—right above his head—as a response to his constant complaints about losing them. And I once dared all of my classmates to sit backward on our chairs before the teacher walked in, just to see the surprised look on his face. Nothing was mean or ill-intentioned, and the harmless pranks brought us together and made us feel good.

I'm sure my parents thought I would outgrow my fondness for practical jokes, but that never quite happened. I have always kept my eyes open for opportunities to have fun. In my twenties, I was on a plane travelling back from a Canada World Youth volunteer trip to Cuba with author (and our late friend) Jacques Hébert; Justin's mom, Margaret Trudeau; and two of his siblings, Sacha (Alexandre) Trudeau and Alicia Kemper. Ally and I spent the first part of the flight watching as an intoxicated man staggered up and down the middle aisle. The flight crew seemed concerned about his behaviour, and I figured I might be able to help. I smiled at him, made a funny comment, and got him engaged in conversation. Then, taking my plan to the next level, I commented on his sunburn and told him about the "best-ever" soothing cream I happened to have in my carry-on. Would he like to try some? I pulled it out, scooped some onto my fingers and, with the man's permission, began to layer it on.

The intoxicated fellow seemed to enjoy the attention, so much so that he didn't notice Ally turning beet red as she tried not to burst out laughing. She'd realized that it wasn't soothing cream I'd been applying to the burnt spots on his face but under-eye concealer, medium-beige tint and full coverage! It showed up as an odd purple-beige on him. Nearby passengers had also picked up on our shenanigans. By the time we were deplaning, and he'd noticed the harmless prank, our formerly disruptive traveller was laughing, too.

A good sense of humour also came in handy the first time I was invited to dinner at Justin's mother's home. I had met Margaret a few times, and we'd hit it off right away. On this particular night, we were all sitting at the dining room table, ready to eat the incredible meal she'd prepared. But just as we were about to begin, a putrid smell filled the room—so strong it actually made me feel nauseated. Because this was my first dinner with the family, I didn't want to make a fuss, but I finally had to say something. "I'm

Only when we are at our most playful can divinity finally get serious with us.

ELIZABETH GILBERT

so sorry," I stammered, "but there is such a bad odour in the air right now that I don't think I can eat." Justin looked at me, puzzled. Margaret seemed surprised. I glanced all around me and then down at the floor. And there, right beside my chair, was a little "gift" from her new and not quite house-trained puppy, Daisy! We all burst into laughter, cleaned up the mess, opened the windows, and proceeded to eat. Talk about setting the tone!

Margaret has an incredible sense of humour, which is why I felt at ease pulling a little prank on her only a few months later. She'd gone to the family cottage in the Laurentian woods with some of her girlfriends, for a getaway weekend, bringing Daisy along. In the middle of their weekend, I called the cottage and pretended to be an employee with the local wildlife organization. When Margaret answered, I disguised my voice, introduced myself as "Caroline SansRegret," and informed her that there was a bear in the area—very, very dangerous. "You must remain inside and close all the curtains and make sure your pets are kept indoors," I said, layering on the details. "The bear is very aggressive and could attack if he sees shadows through the windows."

As a shocked Margaret hung up the phone, I could hear her asking her friends to call Daisy inside right away. A couple of minutes later, Justin (who was in on the prank) got a call on his cellphone from his mom, asking what she should do. Justin suggested that they all take turns standing guard at the front door.

As hard as Justin and I were laughing, I didn't want to ruin Margaret's weekend. I waited an hour and then called the cottage again. In the guise of Caroline SansRegret, I told her that if she needed to go outside to stand watch, she should wear a camouflage coat. I went on to suggest that if she didn't have one, she could call Holt Renfrew and ask to speak to personal shopper Sophie Grégoire, who would help her find something perfect.

There was a long silence on the line, and then I heard: "SOPH! YOU BRAT!"

We all got such a laugh out of it that she included the story in her book *Changing My Mind*. And here it is in mine. Full circle.

Just in case you're wondering, I can take a joke as well as I can dish one out. When Justin and I were dating, a popular Quebec talk show hosted by Véronique Cloutier asked me to come on for an interview. Véronique and I had studied together in CEGEP and had stayed in touch. I'd always liked her, and I admired her hosting skills, humour, and down-to-earth manner. At one point during the interview, she introduced a guest from backstage—a man, she told the audience, who had bad taste in fashion and real trouble dressing for his various commitments. She asked if I'd be willing to help him live on camera. I thought it was a slightly odd request, but I went along with it and took a look at the guy walking toward me. Because I'm near-sighted and have to squint in order to focus when I'm not wearing my glasses, I couldn't see his face well. I noticed only how awkward he looked, with knee-high socks, tight shorts, and a very bizarre hat on his head, which had a propeller on top. "Oh my, what now," I thought to myself. But then I looked closer. It was . . . Justin!

He had agreed to play "bad dress-up" for this skit, and the joke was on me. Oh, did I ever laugh. I also thought it was pretty cool that he didn't give a damn about what people thought. Over the years, he's deliberately fallen on flights of stairs, in hotel lobbies, and down ski hills, just to make me laugh. And even though we are no longer a couple, I know our shared sense of humour will always help us weather the storms.

For me, nothing works as well as a laugh when it comes to forging a connection. Comedian and actor Mark Critch—creator of the comedy TV series *Son of a Critch*—senses this in his work as well. "The best reaction I see in an audience isn't necessarily a laugh, but one person nudging the other, saying, 'That's me!' or 'That's us!'" he told me. "That means you've hit on a truth, and it really connects with them." He also believes there's something magical about hearing a group of people who don't know one another laughing together. "They're all different backgrounds, different colours, different sexes. But they are united in that moment."

On the day I spoke to Mark over Zoom, I was at my desk, in front of my computer. I was totally focused on enjoying our conversation, until, about thirty minutes in, something changed. I kept feeling a weird sensation when I'd shift in my chair. It was as if something pointy was poking me in the butt—something that definitely shouldn't have been there. Not wanting to interrupt the flow of our chat, I subtly felt around, trying to figure out exactly what was going on. And when I finally did, I had to let Mark in on the joke. One of my kids had decided to start our Christmas traditions a bit early and had hidden a surprise under the cushion of my chair. It turned out I was sitting on the Elf on the Shelf's long, pointy nose!

Mark burst into laughter along with me, and then we got back to our very timely conversation about the healing role of humour and laughter for the mind and soul.

Sophie Grégoire: How can we use humour to bring people closer together?

Mark Critch: I think humour is truth, and we laugh at something because we are either shocked by it or we're comforted by it. But it's a shared community. We have to understand the reference, and it's also breaking a pattern, right? Humour and trauma are kind of different paths of the same thing in that a lot of traumatic moments happen when a pattern is broken. And comedy is all about a set-up and then the humorous line breaks the pattern.

263

I always say comedy is the only art form that you can't fake success at. If you're a comedian and people don't laugh—knowing that laughter is involuntary, just like sneezing or vomiting—then you know you're in the wrong.

SG: I was bulimic—I used to vomit when I chose—so I guess I'm the exception to the rule [laughs].

MC: What you just said there—isn't that a way of coping with something? In that moment, we're saying, "Yeah, people might be afraid to say that about themselves, but by doing it, we share a moment." Now we've stepped a little bit closer together. We shared a truth, and comedy is truth, but laughter—you can't really fake an honest laugh.

SG: From a mental health perspective, can humour be used as a validating and reassuring tool?

MC: When someone laughs, they're saying, "Me, too, that happened to me as well. Oh my god." What a comforting thing in life to know that despite all the horrible things that happen in the world and despite the meanness of some people, you get a thousand people in a room together, and when you're laughing, you are defenceless. Stuff is coming out of your nose; you're spitting up a bit; you're bending over. Sometimes people will pee [laughs].

SG: What's that line again? "I was laughing so hard that tears fell down my thighs!" Laughter is also good for our health, isn't it?

MC: [Laughs.] Exactly, right? Yes. It helps with blood circulation; it releases natural painkillers. You get on a natural high that is helpful to you.

SG: Has being a comedian helped you to be a more vulnerable speaker and a more vulnerable and deep listener?

MC: Oh god, yes. Well, a lot of comedy is about listening. Any of the great moments I've had interviewing somebody have come because I was listening. Sometimes through comedy, you're playing like a child would, but you need the other person to dance with you, right? That's a beautiful thing. It's like music and two people singing together. I think to be aware of how people feel about things, or to be aware of disparities, you have to have emotional intelligence. You have to be able to understand. And I think many people with depression or who came from a traumatic childhood have those things because they're hyper-aware of what's happening around them. I think what is noble about being a comedian, or about humour or anything artistic, really, is that you can make people go, "Look, the world can be tough, but the world's beautiful and there's a lot of hope in it, and look what we all just did tonight. Look at the joy we all had. Look, we all came together."

Well, I certainly won't ever have any regrets about making people laugh. If I wasn't able to laugh, and make others around me laugh, too, I think the flame that fuels me would slowly die down. I'm serious. When I play and laugh, I feel so relaxed and deeply connected to myself and others.

Catherine Price is able to explain exactly why we feel so good when we are having fun. Price is an author (*How to Break Up with Your Phone*, *The Power of Fun*, *Vitamania*), an award-winning journalist, and a public speaker. She's studied the positive impacts of playfulness, connection, and flow on our mental and physical health. And she told me that when all three happen at once, that's when we're really having fun.

Sophie Grégoire: What happens from a neurological standpoint when we experience fun?

Catherine Price: There's a lot of research about playfulness and connection and flow being very good states for our feelings of well-being, for our productivity, and for our creativity—the effect that those states can have on our stress hormones.

It's well-known that emotional stress is bad for us over the long-term because it increases our risks for diseases such as heart attack, stroke, dementia, cancer, obesity, type 2 diabetes—the list goes on. And they're all associated with the stress hormone cortisol, which is there to help us flee and survive physical attacks. On the flip side, I don't think most of us recognize that a lack of social connection, or loneliness and isolation, have the same negative effects, because they also increase cortisol levels. It's very important that we feel connected. When you're having fun with someone else, you're not seeing them as someone who's from a different political party or nationality or what have you; you're actually connecting with them as a human being.

If my definition of fun holds true, and it is a state in which you are playful—so you're not taking yourself seriously, you're kind of relaxed, and you're also connected with other people and totally engaged and present—then you're lowering your emotional stress as you connect. You're not lonely when you're having fun. To me, that suggests that in terms of what fun can do to us physiologically, it actually is a health intervention.

SG: As readers of this chapter have discovered, I have a natural sense of "good" mischief in me. I hope that counts as having fun?

CP: One of the themes that stood out to me during my research was of what I call "playful rebellion," but it could also be called mischief or mischievousness. And it was exactly what you're talking about; it was about breaking the rules of adult life just a little bit—not too much, not something totally crazy. For example, I recently met a woman in her forties who showed me pictures of her and her friends, and they had turned one of their basements into a disco roller-skating rink. That's the kind of rebellion I'm talking about. Totally ethical, no one's getting hurt, you're not breaking the law, but you're just doing something a little playfully deviant, and really, that's a very good way to let go in a way that leads to fun. Also, embracing delight (inspired by *The Book of Delights* by Ross Gay) is important. There is evidence behind the idea that noticing positive things in your life, labelling them, and saying them out loud can boost your mood.

SG: The brain is nourished when it's being creative. Have you seen links between playfulness, fun, flow, and creativity?

CP: Yes, flow in particular. To be creative, you need to open yourself and not just shut down ideas before they even have a chance to come forward. When we're having fun, we are being vulnerable, because our walls are down, and that's a very conducive state to creativity. And when you feel connected and safe with people, then you also can allow new ideas to flow.

SG: The multi-tasking, the constant distractions—can we really have fun when we're in these states?

CP: No, you can't, 100 percent no. You have to be in flow to have fun, and anything that distracts you is going to keep you out of flow. By definition, you're not present in your life if you're distracted. The word *distracted* comes from the Latin words for "to drag away," so if your attention is dragged away from something else, you might be physically present, but you are not actually there.

The Comforts of Creativity

When I was six or seven years old, I asked my mother for a book of rhymes and poetry. I think that was when I fell in love with words. They became friends I wanted to hang out with, and I longed to discover their hidden truths. I still do. Language allows us to become more intimate with life and with others. Words carry so much weight that a single sentence can lift you up or pull you down. I started writing early and excelled in my writing classes. When writing birthday cards or thank-you notes, I love playing with words, dancing with them, connecting them to give weight to my emotional message. The late poet Yves Bonnefoy said that "poetry is like trying to encapsulate the intimate silence between the words." I believe that "intimate silence" is where we can meet ourselves and the emotions we carry. It is also where human beings truly meet.

Of course, writing is just one way we can express ourselves. I wasn't the best student in art class at school, but I absolutely loved the deliberate slowness of the creative process, which delights in presence, focus, and attention. I didn't know it then, but I've come to see the creation of anything artistic as a direct pathway to mindfulness and presence. We cannot create if we are distracted or anxious. We must be in the moment, fully engaged in what we are doing. I appreciate that now in a way I was too young to understand as a student, when I was simply enamoured by colours, shapes, lines, and curves. I'll always remember painting a picture of me and my boyfriend horseback riding in Kelowna. As I was working on it, my father would occasionally come and look at my brush strokes. He had never painted, so it was a surprise when he offered some very insightful comments on how to create more light and better contours. I was moved by his sensitive perception and felt, in that moment, connected to him in a way I couldn't explain. It's close to the feeling I get when I'm in the presence of artists—a way of being and of loving life. As Henry Moore said, "To be an artist is to believe in life." I couldn't agree more.

Although I fell in love with painting early, I never thought I was good enough to pursue my own art seriously. I started taking painting lessons only in my forties. Like my eighty-year-old fellow art class student said to me once, "It's never too late, honey!"

The more I paint, the more I believe I can. My painting teacher, David Kearn, says that art begins where judgment ends. I think we could say the same thing of love and of life. Everything becomes more authentic, including ourselves, when we let go of self-criticism and judgment. Creativity is within all of us. We are all artists, in a sense, adding brush strokes to the canvas of our lives every second of every day. We just need to let go of our fear first. In her book *Big Magic: Creative Living Beyond Fear*, Elizabeth Gilbert adopts a great metaphor to describe her evolving relationship with fear and creativity: "I decided that I would need to build an expansive enough interior life that my fear and my creativity could peacefully coexist, since it appeared that they would always be together . . . Fear and creativity shared a womb, they were born at the same time, and they still share some vital organs." Later on, she professes, "I'm on a mission of artistic liberation."

That's exactly how I feel. During the past decades, creativity has taken a technological turn and changed the way we think, work, and play. It's not just about pen on paper anymore. There are so many new ways to create. Our minds had to rewire, and our learning curve grew exponentially. This came with many upsides, but there are downsides, like visual and noise pollution. Whether from drawing apps or creative virtual games, we receive and process news and information at a chaotic speed these days, which disturbs our sensory system and our nervous system. This is why it is so important to take advantage of the comforts that creativity brings, and to remind ourselves that slowing down and being present is an art form in itself.

Dr. Anna Abraham, author of *The Neuroscience of Creativity*, studies the psychological and neurophysiological basis of creativity and other aspects of human imagination. She has described creativity as a state in which we are actually aware of our own unique potential. We talked about the benefits of making room for creativity in our lives.

Sophie Grégoire: What does creativity offer to those willing to embrace it?

Dr. Anna Abraham: What creativity allows is a mirror into what you uniquely are capable of, and that's why it can be a source of strength in times of deprivation and adversity. The strength of expressing and bringing to fruition what only you inherently know can take you places. The creative impulse can make the biggest difference in trying to make something of yourself, or trying to change a reality.

SG: What's the most remarkable thing you've discovered about creativity in human beings and the human brain?

AA: Perhaps the most surprising was what I refer to as the "damage-resistant capacity" of the human brain to be creative. Even with small brain lesions—tiny injuries in the brain—you routinely see huge functions being sort of blanked out. But because creativity is such a complex process involving so many brain systems, it's virtually impossible to snuff out, and that's kind of incredible. This is what makes it possible to use creative techniques in service of rehabilitation.

SG: Is creativity a choice?

AA: Creativity is a fact. We are a creative species, but how we decide to be creative is a choice, and whether we decide to be creative is a choice. We have the capacity to count, but whether we decide to do trigonometry on a daily basis or not is a choice, right?

SG: And when we are being creative, we are using both our left-brain language logic and our right-brain emotions, correct?

AA: Yes, yes, yes! Abundant research has shown us there is no single brain region, no single brain network, no single brain activity patterns that are exclusive for creativity.

SG: Can you explain the distinction between active and passive engagement when it comes to creativity?

AA: We have all these systems in place as markers of a creative moment. The state of flow, for instance, is a well-studied one. Regardless of whether we're talking about an athlete or a painter, the period when they're experiencing their most creative, productive self is usually marked by a sort of flow state, and that's when they're actively engaged in their task and are perfectly aligned in their performance.

But a flow state—at least parts of it—can be passively induced by engaging in tasks that allow you to not track the passage of time or be aware of yourself. So it could be through binge-watching shows, [where] you just get immersed in a completely different stage that mimics some aspects of the flow experience. That's passive interest. It's not creative at all. It doesn't leave you feeling energized, which is very different from what people feel when it's an active interest. So I would definitely distinguish between those two states, an active pursuit of something versus those systems being co-opted in a passive way.

SG: Most people become bored very quickly in our culture. What is the relationship with creativity here?

AA: I actually try to push myself into situations of boredom so that I can let my imagination run wild. I see a lot of positives in encouraging the state of boredom, because you allow your imagination to actively switch on. Usually, boredom is a good place from which to start to change. But if I'm going to be on my phone all the time, listening to a podcast or listening to a song or preoccupied with social media, I'm not really engaging in these imaginative runaway spaces. I think boredom's got a bad rap.

SG: Can creativity help heal trauma?

AA: Creativity can really be conducive to exploring something more intimately, in more detail, in a way that is really personal to you, and a part of [processing] trauma is being able to acknowledge it to yourself. A great example is singer-songwriter Tori Amos, who on her first album talked about her experience of rape in one of the songs, and it's incredibly evocative because she goes through it detail by detail. The word never comes out, but for anyone who has been through that kind of horribly unfortunate situation, hearing that song is revealing, resonating, and can be cathartic.

Speaking through your artwork, regardless of the medium, you're not thinking about who necessarily is engaging with it, and that allows you to really express yourself fully. Through creativity, you are making yourself understood to yourself.

This is quite the reveal. Making yourself seen and known to your own self is a source of freedom. We all want to be free *in* the world, not from it. And humour, playfulness, and creativity can help us get there. They're already within us to discover.

Committing to Creative Fitness
WITH DR. ANNA ABRAHAM

Trying to find a creative outlet can feel overwhelming if you aren't naturally drawn to one type of expression or another. But it's easier than we think, especially if we're willing to commit to creativity the way we are to other things that benefit our health and sense of well-being. Anna Abraham has three tips to get us started:

Anna Abraham: First, think about creativity in terms of a personal pursuit. What tasks help you engage in a process of self-discovery? Some people like to write. Some people like to take photographs. Some people like to experiment in the kitchen. What makes you curious?

The second thing is to think about creativity like your physical fitness or health. Devote time and space to creative fitness in your schedule, because otherwise it's not going to happen.

The third is to not necessarily share it with anyone. Because the minute it becomes about other peoples' eyes, it becomes less about what you want to discover for yourself and more about getting positive regard, which is fine if you're stable enough in your practice to have that. But getting to that space of self-confidence while maintaining your authenticity takes time, experience, and discipline. The main thing is to really enjoy the process of self-discovery.

Ultimately, the most important thing in creativity is to cultivate curiosity about yourself and your mind's powers.

When we try to protect ourselves

from the inevitability of change,

we are not listening to the soul.

To listen to our soul is to slow down,

to feel deeply, to see ourselves clearly,

to surrender to discomfort and

uncertainty and to wait.

ELIZABETH LESSER

Conclusion

Never Strangers

O ne of the most impressive scientific feats of the twenty-first century thus far has come in the field of nuclear energy. Today's nuclear reactors work through *fission*, a process in which a large, unstable atomic nucleus is split into two smaller atoms, releasing energy. It requires a very specific, potentially hazardous element, like uranium, to function. This is just one reason why *fusion* reactors are likely the future of nuclear energy. Instead of separating one large nucleus, fusion reactors merge two smaller ones, and in doing so, release much more energy than fission does.

I'm inspired by this new discovery because of its "green" potential,

> *As your emotional biography sets the musical scale of your life, your unwounded soul writes the ultimate, final symphony.*
>
> SOPHIE GRÉGOIRE TRUDEAU

but I'm also moved by the metaphor it offers us on a human level: we, too, are more powerful when we come together and work together. When we are conscious of and understand our own emotional patterns, we are able to offer compassion to ourselves and others. This is the starting place from which we can foster a true sense of togetherness and community, and create hope for the present and the future. But to do so means committing to the work required to connect with our authentic selves. Somehow, in our hurry to become adults and accomplish our life goals, we forget how essential it is to stay connected to the legitimate needs of the child within us. We might not be that child anymore, but as we've seen, we still carry with us the wiring and insecurities of our childhood.

One thing that comes to mind (no pun intended) when we think about the never-ending quest to understand how we human beings work is that our brain is a relational organ. From cradle to grave, we grow, we love, we suffer, we retract, we connect, we evolve, and we live in relationship to others and the world around us—all while our brains anticipate and register every single moment of interaction. As Dr. Georg Northoff—neuroscientist, author, philosopher, psychiatrist, and head of the Royal's Institute of Mental Health Research in Ottawa—told me: "The better alignment between our mind-brain and the environment, the more we feel in the 'groove.'" (I can hear the chorus of Madonna's "Into the Groove" right now.)

In simple terms, the degree of synchrony between yourself and your surroundings determines the quality of your neurological processes. As Georg explained, "a great part of the promising future of mental health and psychiatry will depend on our capacity to bring the 'time' of the brain into synchrony with 'real time,' since mental disorders are basically a source of misalignment between the respective

276

bodily and environmental context. This, in turn, disorganizes our experiences and our consciousness in spatial and temporal terms."

The wording here may be quite scientific, but it's absolutely fascinating to comprehend how our brain's constant search for synchrony and alignment with our body and our environment is a double-edged sword. On one side, it allows us to remain stable and able to experience life. On the other, it makes us vulnerable to life events that can disturb that relationship. As we know, traumatic events can lead to post-traumatic disorders, and Dr. Northoff's group and research show that "the time perception of subjects with high degrees of early childhood traumatic life events is more disrupted and less continuous, leading to high degrees of depression."

The great news is that there are simple healing tools being developed. From brain-based meditation to help reduce speed of thought and anxiety to music therapy, connecting with nature, and transcranial stimulation, the well-being of our brains is at the core of how we can influence and help build a better future.

The time and patience and psychological flexibility required to recognize my emotional patterns didn't come naturally to me, but I know why now. That was my lesson. And it still is. I'm a giver, a doer. Well, you can't get time and patience "done." It's more like they do you. Slowing down comes with the responsibility of looking at life and ourselves consciously—straight up, as is.

It also means not being afraid to come closer together as we build stronger and more authentic relationships. Governor General Mary Simon confided, "When I first got appointed as governor general, I set up some priorities, and two of them were reconciliation [between Indigenous peoples and other Canadians] and mental health. How do I address reconciliation? I thought about it a lot, talked to people, and what it really is, is for me to be sitting here with you right now, telling my story. So that you understand who I am and you, in turn, can tell me your story, and therefore a bond can be reached. Now that can be multiplied hundreds of thousands of millions of times just by doing those types of good acts."

Her Excellency's words apply to the work that needs to take place in Canada, but they can also apply to all communities in which differences need to be reconciled. Sitting together as people of the same planet can get complicated, in practice, if we forget how intertwined we are. On a parallel note, Dr. Carol Hopkins, chief executive officer of the Thunderbird Partnership Foundation, reminds us that Western culture has so much to learn from the holistic view of Indigenous knowledge when it comes to well-being. She speaks of wellness as a balance between the four aspects of our being—spirit, emotions, mind, body. "An Indigenous world view holds spirit as central to all life, and therefore central to wellness," she told me. And yet "the very idea that we, as people, have a 'relationship' with the earth and all beings that live on the earth is a foreign concept in the theoretical models that inform mental health. 'Holistic' is a value that promotes interconnectedness and interdependence."

Now we know that this concept of interdependence is relevant not only from a spiritual perspective but also from a biological imperative. We are stronger, in so many ways, when we come together.

Something positive takes place in our brains when we commit to self-inquiry *and* connection with others. It reminds me of how author Martha Beck (*The Way of Integrity*) speaks of the neurology of awakening. According to one study, inquiry and self-contemplation turn a temporary brain *state* of unity and love into a permanent, structural brain *trait*. This is how much atomic power our habits can create!

In my late thirties, I really wanted to dig into my own patterns, and I had deep discussions on the topic with an insightful mentor. At one point during our work, he confided that he'd had a serious mouth surgery and was having enunciation problems as a result. And so, for months, we conducted our sessions via Skype, where I would talk and he would type his responses. It was a unique exchange, demanding I slow down and pay extra attention to these written answers so as not to miss anything. After a break over the summer months, I learned that my guiding friend had died. I was in pain, but I knew that, finally, his pain was gone. To this day, I still feel his spiritual presence. He once dared me to sing to him over the phone, which I did (a song I had written for Ella-Grace called "Smile Back at Me"). Weeks after his passing, I found the only poem he'd ever sent my way. I share part of it with you here because it resonates with me now more than ever, and reminds me that when we move in synchronicity with the rhythm of life, nothing is missing. We are whole, and our hearts, minds, and bodies sing to each other.

> you are full of light
> full of love
> and real strength
> gifts
> to receive
> and give again
>
> in this work
> that is the melody
> of really living
> we feel called
> to free our gifts
> we follow that call
> and discover
> all we need to do
> is simply free ourselves
>
> from this point of freedom
> it all expresses
> like the sun
> a point of light
> expressing so many unique rays

soulful

homecoming

really being with all we are and were

the light the dark

the welcomed parts

the banished parts

of ourselves

behind all the jazz

this is the reality that everyone is living

and as you decode this in yourself

as you embrace it all

all of Her

you finally decode

finally embrace

everyone else

their hearts suddenly known to you

by setting yourself free

you set others free

which means

all you have to do is dance

your dance

and all else will follow

. . .

welcome home . . .

The more we feel at home within ourselves, the better our chances to build a safe emotional home out there in the world. The quality and clarity of our thoughts and emotions will shape our shared future and our mental well-being.

I do hope what you've read in these pages helps you feel more at home with yourself. Finding your safe, calm, and creative self is the starting place for all that follows, and the loving relationship you develop and nourish with yourself is the most important one you'll ever be in. Our task is to build intimacy with what and who makes us feel whole and encourages our growth as we dare to unearth our own true self.

Now, let's resist the urge to skip this:

Inhale courage . . .
Exhale all of your doubts . . .
Inhale tenderness . . .
Exhale all your rigid parts . . .
Inhale peace . . .
Exhale patience . . .

It might seem like we're reaching an end together, but I see it as a new beginning—from this point of stillness where you are alive, and whole, and safe. Like a baby who explores its surroundings in part through falling and getting back up, again and again, we, too, will trip up on occasion. That's life. But the next time you fall, know that I'd hold out a helping hand, and maybe share a couple of giggles to make you smile. And what if we all did that for each other? We can help each other get back up. There is no wealth of being without mental wealth! In this way, we can lead an emotional revolution for the sake of our own evolution.

From beginning to end, we are never strangers. Let us come closer together. I hope to meet you on the path.

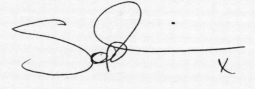

Acknowledgements

When I read a book, I sometimes skip over the acknowledgements. But each time, I catch myself and wonder why. These pages often tell us about the author's sense of gratitude, about how the story came alive, and about who contributed to it. Now that I'm writing my own acknowledgements, I know how important it is to share this information and honour those who have helped along the way.

About twelve years ago, I read a book called *In the Realm of Hungry Ghosts* by Dr. Gabor Maté. The content moved me so profoundly that I looked deeper into the work of this addiction specialist. More than a decade later, and twenty years into my mental health advocacy work, a helpful friend suggested I meet with Gabor while he was giving a talk in Ottawa. My first thought was "Why would he ever want to meet with me? He's such a busy man." Thankfully, he was aware of my volunteer activism and took the time to get together. And when I asked him to, he looked at an early outline for this book. Thank you, G, for helping me on this path, and to connect with a community of experts who, in my mind, are insightful and powerful peacemakers. I will not forget how the sun was shining on that fall day. It felt like it was conspiring in our favour.

To the team of strong and courageous women at Random House—Sue Kuruvilla, Pamela Murray, Deirdre Molina, Lisa Jager, Catherine Abes, Christie Hanson, Erin Cooper, Kristin Cochrane, Marion Garner, Beth Lockley, Anaïs Loewen-Young, Danielle LeSage, and Adrienne Tang—and you, too, Evan Klein: What an incredible group you are. Thank you for your trust in me, but most of all, thank you for knowing the responsibility we all hold in making the world a better place and how we should all have each other's backs, hearts, and minds!

To my editor and "all day, all evening, weekends included" invaluable collaborator Linda Pruessen: the late phone calls, the incessant work in such a crunched period of time, the little moments of panic, and the ones filled with laughter and hope, thank you for your clarity of thought, kindness of heart, and brilliance of mind.

To copy editor Stacey Cameron and proofreader Sue Sumeraj: thank you for your sharp eyes—life is in the details!

Thank you to Angelika Heim and my allies Thomas Laporte Aust and Jody Colero for your guidance, vision, and friendship.

To the wellness, yoga, or meditation teachers I've studied or taught with: You have infused my life, my body, and my mind with more wisdom and self-awareness. Thank you, Barrie, Mona, Robin, Natalie, Louise, Tracy, Ryan, Sylvie, Travis and Lauren, my friend Andrea, and the whole yoga community, wherever you are in this world, practising and teaching integrity of movement, thought, and action.

To all my favourite colleagues and collaborators: Thank you for the support you have shown me and my family through the years.

I couldn't have done it all without you: Dunerci, Sarah, John, Coral, and the whole incredible "24" family. Eddie, Laura, Annie, and all others who helped me look after my well-being. To every RCMP member who has shown me and my family warmth, a caring attitude, and professionalism. It has been an honour to share our days with you.

To my true best friends, circle of sisters, and beloved uncles and cousins: You (obviously) know who you are. What a big and tight family we form. Many of you have seen me in front of my computer or carrying my laptop like a baby in a sling for months, and you witnessed how learning more and writing about such a universal topic made me profoundly happy. I was blessed with your patience and kindness. My "giant rock": the love we share every day makes me feel seen, validated, safe, and understood.

To my parents, Estelle and Jean, I love you. I know you did your best, traversing your own emotional journeys, at every step. I'm eternally grateful for the life you gave me. To my mother-in-law, Margaret, I'm grateful for our friendship and I admire the courage you've shown in sharing your own mental-health journey.

To my family and kids, Xavier, Ella-Grace, and Hadrien. You are my well of love. My source of inspiration. Now and forever. To Justin: sharing life, parenting, and raising incredible kids together has been the most beautiful adventure. We will always navigate the waters of our bond with respect, care, friendship, and love.

And to you, dear reader, whether we have met or not, all I can say is: "I loved you first . . ."

Further Reading

Brewer, Judson. *The Craving Mind: From Cigarettes to Smartphones to Love—Why We Get Hooked & How We Can Break Bad Habits.* New Haven, CT: Yale University Press, 2018.

———. *Unwinding Anxiety: New Science Shows How to Break the Cycles of Worry and Fear to Heal Your Mind.* New York: Penguin Random House, 2022.

Campbell, Susan, and John Grey. *Five-Minute Relationship Repair: Quickly Heal Upsets, Deepen Intimacy, and Use Differences to Strengthen Love.* Novato, CA: New World Library, 2015.

Comella, Lynn. *Vibrator Nation: How Feminist Sex-Toy Stores Changed the*

Business of Pleasure. Durham, NC: Duke University Press, 2017.

Dana, Deb. *Anchored: How to Befriend Your Nervous System Using Polyvagal Theory.* Sounds True, 2021.

——. *Polyvagal Exercises for Safety and Connection: 50 Client-Centered Practices.* New York: W. W. Norton, 2020.

Dweck, Carol. *Mindset: The New Psychology of Success.* New York: Ballantine Books, 2016.

Gilbert, Elizabeth. *Big Magic: Creative Living Beyond Fear.* New York: Riverhead Books, 2022.

Heisz, Jennifer. *Move the Body, Heal the Mind: Overcome Anxiety, Depression, and Dementia and Improve Focus, Creativity, and Sleep.* New York: HarperCollins, 2016.

Hendrix, Harville, and Helen LaKelly Hunt. *Getting the Love You Want: A Guide for Couples*, 3rd ed. New York: St. Martin's Griffin, 2019.

Kang, Shimi. *The Dolphin Parent: A Guide to Raising Healthy, Happy, and Self-Motivated Kids.* Toronto: Penguin Canada, 2015.

——. *The Tech Solution: Creating Healthy Habits for Kids Growing Up in a Digital World.* Toronto: Penguin Canada, 2020.

Kaplan, Bonnie J., and Julia J. Rucklidge. *The Better Brain: Overcome Anxiety, Combat Depression, and Reduce ADHD and Stress with Nutrition.* New York: HarperCollins, 2021.

Lembke, Anna. *Dopamine Nation: Finding Balance in the Age of Indulgence.* New York: Penguin Random House, 2021.

Léonard. Stéphanie. *Miroir miroir: Vivre avec son corps.* Montreal: Semaine, 2015.

Levine, Amir, and Rachel S. F. Heller. *Attached: The New Science of Adult Attachment and How It Can Help You Find—and Keep—Love.* New York: Penguin, 2012.

Maté, Gabor. *In the Realm of Hungry Ghosts: Close Encounters with Addiction.* Toronto: Knopf Canada, 2008.

——. *The Myth of Normal: Trauma, Illness & Healing in a Toxic Culture.* Toronto: Knopf Canada, 2022.

——. *When the Body Says No: The Cost of Hidden Stress.* Toronto: Vintage Canada, 2021.

Nay, W. Robert. *Taking Charge of Anger: Six Steps to Asserting Yourself Without Losing Control*, 2nd ed. New York: Guilford Press, 2012.

Neufeld, Gordon, and Gabor Maté. *Hold On to Your Kids: Why Parents Need to Matter More than Peers*. Toronto: Vintage, 2013.

Perel, Esther. *Mating in Captivity: Unlocking Erotic Intelligence*. New York: HarperCollins, 2006.

Pharaon, Vienna. *The Origins of You: How Breaking Family Patterns Can Liberate the Way We Live and Love*. New York: G. P. Putnam's Sons, 2023.

Plank, Liz. *For the Love of Men: From Toxic to a More Mindful Masculinity*. New York: St. Martin's Griffin, 2021.

Pollan, Michael. *The Omnivore's Dilemma: A Natural History of Four Meals*. New York: Penguin Books, 2007.

Porges, Stephen. *The Pocket Guide to the Polyvagal Theory: The Transformative Power of Feeling Safe*. New York: W. W. Norton, 2017.

Price, Catherine. *How to Break Up with Your Phone: The 30-Day Plan to Take Back Your Life*. New York: Ten Speed Press, 2018.

———. *The Power of Fun: How to Feel Alive Again*. New York: Dial Press, 2021.

Real, Terrence. *I Don't Want to Talk about It: Overcoming the Secret Legacy of Male Depression*. New York: Scribner, 1998.

———. *The New Rules of Marriage: What You Need to Know to Make Love Work*. New York: Ballantine Books, 2008.

———. *Us: Getting Past You & Me to Build a More Loving Relationship*. New York: Rodale, 2022.

Siegel, Daniel. *IntraConnected: MWe (Me + We) as the Integration of Self, Identity, and Belonging*. New York: Norton Professional Books, 2022.

Smith, David Livingstone. *Less than Human: Why We Demean, Enslave, and Exterminate Others*. New York: St. Martin's Griffin, 2012.

———. *Making Monsters: The Uncanny Power of Dehumanization*. Cambridge, MA: Harvard University Press, 2021.

———. *On Inhumanity: Dehumanization and How to Resist It*. New York: Oxford University Press, 2020.

Swingle, Mari K. *i-Minds: How and Why Constant Connectivity Is Rewiring Our Brains and What to Do about It*, 2nd ed. Gabriola Island, BC: New Society, 2019.

Tsabary, Shefali. *The Awakened Family: How to Raise Empowered, Resilient, and Conscious Children.* New York: Penguin, 2017.

———. *The Conscious Parent: Transforming Ourselves, Empowering Our Children.* Vancouver, BC: Namaste Publishing, 2010.

———. *The Parenting Map: Step-by-Step Solutions to Consciously Create the Ultimate Parent-Child Relationship.* New York: HarperCollins, 2023.

Zolotow, Nina. *Yoga for Times of Change: Practices and Meditations for Moving through Stress, Anxiety, Grief & Life's Transitions.* Boulder, CO: Shambhala, 2022.

Selected Notes

Introduction

Jamie Ducharme, "The Happiness Professor Takes Her Own Advice," *Time*,
    January 16, 2023.

World Health Organization, "Mental Disorders," June 8, 2022.
    https://www.who.int/news-room/fact-sheets/detail/mental-disorders.

Esther Perel, LinkedIn, 2022. https://www.linkedin.com/posts/estherperel_the
    -quality-of-our-relationships-determines-activity-68635621242287975424
    -9LJe/.

Chapter 1

Jennifer Paris, Antoinette Ricardo, Dawn Rymond, and Alexa Johnson, *Child Growth and Development*, ed. 1.2 (Santa Clarita, CA: College of the Canyons, 2019). https://open.umn.edu/opentextbooks/textbooks/750.

Chapter 2

Kasee Bailey, "Five Powerful Health Benefits of Journaling," Intermountain Health Care, July 31, 2018. https://intermountainhealthcare.org/blogs /topics/live-well/2018/07/5-powerful-health-benefits-of-journaling/.

Chapter 3

V. Franchina and G. Lo Coco, "The Influence of Social Media Use on Body Image Concerns," *International Journal of Psychoanalysis and Education* 10, no. 1 (2018): 5–14.

J. Fardouly and L. R. Vartanian, "Social Media and Body Image Concerns: Current Research and Future Directions," *Current Opinion in Psychology* 9 (2016): 1–5.

G. Holland and M. Tiggemann, "A Systematic Review of the Impact of the Use of Social Networking Sites on Body Image and Disordered Eating Outcomes," *Body Image* 17 (2016): 100–110.

R. Cohen and A. Blaszczynski, "Comparative Effects of Facebook and Conventional Media on Body Image Dissatisfaction," *Journal of Eating Disorders* 3, no. 23 (2015): 1–27.

R. Bachner-Melman, E. Zontag-Oren, A. H. Zohar, and H. Sher, "Lives on the Line: The Online Lives of Girls and Women with and without a Lifetime Eating Disorder Diagnosis," *Frontiers in Psychology* 9 (2018): 1–10.

Tracy Moore, "What Do Men Want?" Jezebel, April 29, 2015. https://jezebel.com /what-do-men-want-obedient-wives-and-independent-daught -1700743721.

"Anorexia Nervosa," Johns Hopkins, n.d. https://www.hopkinsmedicine
.org/health/conditions-and-diseases/eating-disorders/anorexia
-nervosa.

Chapter 4

Tyler Knott Gregson, "When We Are Legend," *Signal Fire*, February 12, 2023.
Maggie Wooll, "Change Your Life (for Good) with More Purpose and
Passion," BetterUp, July 14, 2022. https://www.betterup.com/blog/purpose
-vs-passion.

Chapter 5

Scott Edwards, "On the Brain: Love and the Brain," Harvard Medical School,
Spring 2015. https://hms.harvard.edu/news-events/publications-archive
/on-the-brain.

Chapter 6

"11 Positive Parenting Strategies You Need to Start Using," Prodigy Education,
November 6, 2020. https://www.prodigygame.com/main-en/blog
/positive-parenting/.

Chapter 7

Hadley Leggett, "'Cyclic Sighing' Can Help Breathe Away Anxiety," Scope,
February 9, 2023. https://scopeblog.stanford.edu/2023/02/09/cyclic
-sighing-can-help-breathe-away-anxiety/.
Kirsten Weir, "Nurtured by Nature," American Psychological Association,
April 1, 2020. https://www.apa.org/monitor/2020/04/nurtured-nature.

"Into the Wild: 8 Ways Exercising in Nature Brings Health Benefits,"
Conscious Spaces, July 28, 2021. https://consciousspaces.com/blogs
/science/into-the-wild-8-ways-exercising-in-nature-brings-added
-health-benefits/.

CAMH News and Stories, "Mental Illness Associated with Poor Sleep Quality
According to Largest Study of Its Kind," Canadian Association for Mental
Health, October 12, 2021. https://www.camh.ca/en/camh-news-and-stories
/mental-illness-associated-with-poor-sleep-quality.

Sarah Berger, "Early Birds vs. Night Owls: How One Has an Advantage at Work,
According to Science," CNBC, February 15, 2019. https://www.cnbc.com
/2019/02/15/study-reveals-if-night-or-morning-people-have-brain
-function-advantage.html.

Chapter 8

Esalen Team, "A Conversation with Jewel," Esalen, January 1, 2017.
https://www.esalen.org/post/a-conversation-with-jewel.

Ilana Kaplan, "Jewel Wants You to Be Present," *The New York Times*,
September 30, 2020. https://www.nytimes.com/2020/09/30/style
/jewel-wants-you-to-be-present.html.

"Substance Use and Addiction," Canadian Mental Health Association, n.d.
https://ontario.cmha.ca/addiction-and-substance-use-and-addiction/.

Tom Valentino, "46.3 Million in US Met Criteria for SUD Diagnosis in
2021," Addiction Professional, January 6, 2023. https://www
.hmpgloballearningnetwork.com/site/ap/news/463-million-us-met
-criteria-sud-diagnosis-2021.

Chapter 9

"Mental Health: Anxiety Disorders," Government of Canada, n.d.
https://www.canada.ca/en/health-canada/services/healthy-living
/your-health/diseases/mental-health-anxiety-disorders.html.

"Anxiety Disorders," National Alliance on Mental Illness, December 2017.
     https://www.nami.org/About-Mental-Illness/Mental-Health-Conditions
     /Anxiety-Disorders.
"The Power of the Vagus Nerve," Highpoint Mind & Movement, n.d.
     https://www.highpointaz.com/christinas-blog/the-power-of-the-vagus
     -nerve.
Davide Casiraghi, "Polyvagal Theory for Dummies," Movement Meets Life,
     October 13, 2019. https://www.movementmeetslife.com/en/posts
     /polyvagal-theory-for-dummies.

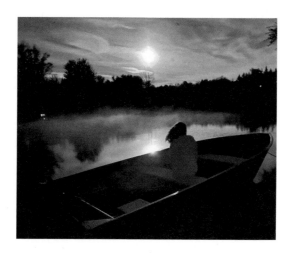

SOPHIE GRÉGOIRE TRUDEAU is an engaged advocate for mental health, emotional literacy, and gender equality. She is a mother of three and an adventurous sportswoman. Over the past twenty years, she has been involved with a variety of causes as a speaker, interviewer, and mentor, including teenage self-esteem, women's and girls' rights and freedoms, and eating disorders. As part of her advocacy work, she shares her time with a number of charities and non-profit organizations. She is the national volunteer for the Canadian Mental Health Association and is Plan International's Youth Leadership Global Ambassador. She is a recipient of the 2013 UN Women National Committee Canada Recognition Award for her contribution to human rights, the 100th Member of Nature Canada's Women for Nature initiative, and a recipient of the Because Mothers Matter Award.

Fully bilingual (and with intermediate Spanish), Sophie studied commerce at McGill University and finished her BA in communications at the Université de Montréal. She completed another degree at the École de radio et de télévision Promédia in Montreal. After her studies, she worked in sales, advertising, and in a newsroom before becoming a television and radio host.

Passionate about movement, exercise, and yoga, Sophie completed both her hatha yoga and "Radiant Child" teacher certifications. She has taught yoga and meditation classes online as well as in different public schools close to her home. She loves painting, writing, playing music, and, most of all, human mischief.